Governing the Crisis

This book presents a multidimensional approach to understanding the effects of COVID-19 on the lifeworld of the marginalised communities in India. The essays in the volume pursue two interrelated concerns: First, they examine the governance aspect, highlighting institutional failures, a lack of political will, and ideological warfare; second, they firmly position the crisis—as a narrative tool—at the heart of marginality, thereby explaining the effects of COVID-19 on communities that continue to remain at the nation's margins. The volume presents varied voices and granular narratives of sufferings that structured the lives of the poorest and dispossessed in the country during the crisis. It dovetails the reshaping of material forces that were crucially impacted by the failure of governance with the social lifeworld of those containing what can be referred to as intergenerational trauma. This volume offers a robust account of the crisis by combining these two distinct but complementary dimensions of COVID-19 in India.

The volume will greatly interest scholars and researchers in crisis studies, governance, medical anthropology, public policy, politics, sociology, and South Asian studies.

Dr Rahul Ranjan is writer and Lecturer (Assistant Professor) in Environmental and Climate Justice at the Department of Human Geography, School of Geosciences, University of Edinburgh. He is the author of *The Political Life of Memory: Birsa Munda in Contemporary India*, which was published by the Cambridge University Press in 2023 and has edited a volume, "*At the crossroads of Rights*", published by Routledge Press, London, 2022. Between 2020 and 2023, he held an appointment as a Postdoctoral Research Fellow to work on the project: *Riverine Rights: The Currents and Consequences of Legal Innovations on the Rights of Rivers*, funded by the Norwegian Research Council in Oslo, Norway.

Governing the Crisis

Narratives of COVID-19 in India

Edited by Rahul Ranjan

Routledge
Taylor & Francis Group
LONDON AND NEW YORK

First published 2025
by Routledge
4 Park Square, Milton Park, Abingdon, Oxon OX14 4RN

and by Routledge
605 Third Avenue, New York, NY 10158

Routledge is an imprint of the Taylor & Francis Group, an informa business

British Library Cataloguing-in-Publication Data
A catalogue record for this book is available from the British Library

ISBN: 978-1-032-45807-6 (hbk)
ISBN: 978-1-032-96998-5 (pbk)
ISBN: 978-1-003-59164-1 (ebk)

DOI: 10.4324/9781003591641

Typeset in Sabon LT Pro
by Apex CoVantage, LLC

Contents

Figures

Tables

Acknowledgements

This volume is a result of collective endeavour. Conceived through months of coordination, workshop, discussions, delays, promises, and the exchange of countless emails, it has finally taken its present form. The envisioning of a workshop without funding is a daunting task, and thus, I am profoundly grateful to the "AsiaNet" forum at the University of Oslo for awarding the International Academic Networking grant during my tenure as a Postdoc in Oslo. This grant facilitated my collaboration with Afreen Gani Faridi, the co-organizer of the "Covid at the Margin" workshop at JKLU University, Jaipur, India. Afreen's unwavering support and meticulous attention to detail were instrumental in the success of our two-day event. Our shared hopes and challenges in this partnership are woven into our joint effort to write, think, and imagine a better, more just world.

Each workshop participant, whether attending in person or online from around the globe, contributed significantly with their insights from the research. Writing, indeed, is never a solitary pursuit. This volume was envisioned during my early days as a postdoc in Oslo and the work continued through to its advanced stage here in Edinburgh, where I teach and research. For this, I am deeply indebted to Kenneth Bo Nielsen, who has continually supported me in various capacities as a mentor and friend.

I am also grateful to my dear friends—Palak Rao, Sebastian Lam, Pulkit Dewan, Ankita Bhartwal, Palak Dudani, Andrea Nightingale, and Ursula Munster—who have provided indispensable support at various stages of this journey. This volume represents a collective effort towards thorough, rich, and empirically grounded scholarship, shedding light on how the pandemic has exacerbated long-standing inequalities in India. May this work highlight the scholarship needed to render grief visible that repletes lives of those who survived and lost.

Contributors

Dr. Aparna Agarwal is Assistant Professor in the School of Government and Public Policy, O.P. Jindal Global University. She is currently pursuing her postdoctoral research as Swiss Government Excellence Fellow at the University of Lausanne. She completed her DPhil from the Department of International Development, University of Oxford. Aparna's DPhil thesis titled "(Re)moving Waste: Caste, Spaces, and Materials in Delhi" examines geographies of waste in relation with the ongoing waste crisis and changing social relations among sanitation and waste workers in Delhi. Her research interests lie in the fields of urban sociology, waste studies, labour studies, anti-caste studies, political ecology, and Indian politics. She is currently working on perceptions of environment around waste sites in Delhi.

Afreen G. Faridi is ICSSR Doctoral Fellow at the Centre for the Study of Law and Governance, Jawaharlal Nehru University, New Delhi, and Assistant Professor of Communication and Critical Thinking at JK Lakshmipat University, Jaipur. He specializes in utilizing political economy to analyse Constitutionalism, Public Policy, and shifts in Labour Practices amongst pastoral tribes of Jammu and Kashmir. His writings include poetry on conflict, trauma, and memory. Afreen founded the Pastoral and Himalayan Academic Network (@Pahad_JK on X) to strengthen grassroot academic capacities in Jammu and Kashmir. Afreen believes that a well-cooked meal can be a potent challenge to bigotry and that a heartfelt poem can be a good tool for introspection.

Rashmi Kumari is a PhD candidate in the Department of Childhood Studies at Rutgers University. Rashmi's doctoral dissertation is an ethnographic study of how development and violence mark the lives of Indigenous children and youth in India. Her research interests are at the intersections of temporalities of childhoods, indigeneity, gender, and political violence.

Dr Pratik Mishra is currently a postdoctoral research assistant with the Oppressive Heat project at Royal Holloway, University of London, and is soon to join as a British Academy Postdoctoral Fellow at the University of Sussex. He is a human geographer whose research looks at different facets of informal labour in the global South including circular migration, worksite-based social reproduction, climate precarity, and social difference. His doctoral research at King's College London concerned the everyday politics of labour within a brick kiln cluster near Delhi, drawing connections between the fields of labour studies, political ecology, and urban studies. He also conducted post-doctoral research on the history of manual scavenging labour in South Asia, looking at caste, coloniality, and urban infrastructure. He is also presently involved in a film-making project on the lifeworlds of brick kiln workers.

Dr Rituparna Patgiri is Assistant Professor of Sociology in the Department of Humanities and Social Sciences (HSS), Indian Institute of Technology (IIT), Guwahati. Her research interests lie in exploring questions of culture, food, media, gender, and pedagogy. Patgiri is one of the co-founders of Doing Sociology—an academic blog dedicated to promoting sociological consciousness among young scholars. At present, she is also serving as the Associate Editor of the South Asian Region in Society—a journal published by Springer Nature that explores the latest scholarship on the central questions of contemporary society.

Ritwika Patgiri is a doctoral researcher in the Faculty of Economics at South Asian University (SAU), New Delhi. She has a master's degree in Economics from Jamia Millia Islamia, New Delhi, and a BA in Economics from Shri Ram College of Commerce, University of Delhi. Her PhD is on Rural Transformation and the Non-Farm Sector in Assam. She has previously worked with The Himalaya Collective, an open-source platform for individuals and organisations living and working in the Himalayan states of Uttarakhand, Himachal Pradesh, and Jammu and Kashmir. Patgiri was the coordinator of the Western Himalayan Vikalp Sangam and looked over the coordination of the various Western Himalayan organisations, documentation of work, drafting of policy briefs, and compilation of the report "Extraordinary Stories of Ordinary People: Pandemic Resilience in the Western Himalayas". She has also received the Zubaan-Sasakawa Peace Foundation Grants for Young Researchers from the Northeast for 2020–2021. Her research interests include rural transformation, migration, poverty, inequality, and feminist economics.

Dr. Manjesh Rana, with a PhD in law, specializes in electoral politics and public policy. He is currently a Senior Program Officer for the International Election Observation Mission Program at the Asian Network for Free Elections (ANFREL) in Thailand. Previously, Dr. Rana served as a public policy fellow at the Delhi Legislative Assembly and worked with Lokniti at the Centre for the Study of Developing Societies (CSDS), where he led significant studies on policing and elections. He also served as Assistant Professor, teaching Constitutional Law at the University of Delhi for over three years. Dr. Rana is dedicated to advancing democratic practices and empowering marginalised communities through his research and advocacy.

Nishant Sirohi is a Health & Human Rights Fellow at Geneva Health Files (Switzerland) and a Law & Society Fellow at Transitions Research, Goa (India). His research focuses on the relationship between human rights and development—issues related to social inequalities, environment, and health. Nishant holds an MPhil in Theory and Practice of Human Rights from the University of Oslo (Norway) and a BA LLB (Hons) degree from Aligarh Muslim University (India).

Sushmita is an international award-winning journalist, researcher, photographer, and former engineer. She has worked on issues of environmental justice, forest governance, health, gender, and more. She is a Pulitzer Center grantee, Society for Environmental journalists' diversity fellow, 2024, and winner of Covering Climate Now awards 2024 and Red Ink Awards for excellence in Indian Journalism, 2022. She is a guest lecturer at TISS, Mumbai, where she teaches modules on climate change and health for master's students of public and mental health. Her articles have appeared in India's leading newspapers and magazines and she has won multiple awards for journalistic excellence.

Dr. Aashish Xaxa is Assistant Professor of Sociology, Adivasi/Indigenous Peoples and Development Studies, in the Department of Humanities and Social Sciences, IIT Gandhinagar. He obtained his PhD in Development Studies from the Tata Institute of Social Sciences (TISS), Mumbai, in 2021, where he was an ICSSR Doctoral Fellow. His broader research is on the urbanisation and changing Cityscapes of India, focusing on unexplored aspects of indigeneity, equity, governance, and social justice. He is passionate about decolonial movements around the world, novels, photography, music, and Western Cinema, COVID-19 and the Indigenous migrants' question in urban India.

Foreword

My conversations with Rahul Ranjan about COVID-19 are almost as old as our friendship. I first met Rahul in person at SOAS in London on March 6, 2020, where I was supposed to give a talk at an evening seminar, having returned from India to my hometown of Oslo just a week and a half earlier. There had been some talk in India about a new virus spreading from China, and as I recall, there was some thermal screening of arrivals from select destinations at Dabolim Airport, where I both landed and departed, although activities at the airport otherwise seemed to largely resemble business as usual.

During our stay in India, few people had spoken about "corona". But at Heathrow in early March, things appeared more chaotic. Concerns about the new virus, as we mostly called it, meant that some new measures had been introduced. As far as I remember, there were posters with health information, alongside special instructions to travellers about how to detect and act on possible symptoms; travellers returning from those parts of Italy that had witnessed the first outbreak of the virus in Europe were singled out in particular. But there was no social distancing; no lockdown; no facemasks; and as of yet no stories of loss and suffering, death and mourning. At the bar in the evening, after the seminar had been concluded, we could still joke that we would, as busy academics, actually welcome some extended "corona lockdown time" with not-so-covert references to the famed Mexican beer.

Just a few days later, Rahul returned the visit and came to Oslo to give a talk on Adivasi resistance and memory politics. But even if merely some days had passed since we had said goodbye in London, things had significantly changed. People were jittery and anxious, unsure of what might happen next but anticipating that things might soon move from bad to worse. And yet, hardly anyone had a clear idea of what to expect. There was talk about impending government action involving the introduction of "restrictions" of sorts, and perhaps a lockdown, but this was all still in the realm of speculation when Rahul presented his paper on March 10. Two days later, the Norwegian government announced the introduction of the most far-reaching restrictions ever seen in peaceful times, which were to be implemented with almost immediate effect. Rahul's plane from Gardermoen Airport back to London was among the last to depart before regular air travel was suspended.

The foundation-shaking feeling of uncertainty and anxiety that accompanied the arrival of COVID-19 was intense and inescapable. It was also almost universal in the sense that the very rapid spread of the virus posed an extremely rare and globally synchronised existential challenge that forced humanity across continents and across all categories of social location to confront the same phenomenon, at the same time, with the cognitive, emotional, institutional, social, and political tools at their disposal. Yet if the subjective and existential initial encounter with COVID-19 thus amounted to a virtually universal human experience, the experience with living with and through a prolonged pandemic spanning several years was certainly far from universal. I was reminded of this at a recent and very informal summer party at my local badminton club, where the conversation at one point casually strayed to the theme of COVID-19. "It feels like ages ago" was a common refrain, followed by an assertion that "those were strange days indeed". People reminisced about how, in the spring of 2020, public discussions treated COVID-19 as a game-changer, a radical rupture that would mean that things would never be the same again. But now, with the benefit of hindsight, it seemed to have been a mere parenthesis in our lives, nothing more than a temporary and relatively short-lived interruption of business as usual.

There is, of course, nothing "universal" about this kind of informal conversation in the sense that the COVID experience it articulates is far from generalisable. Indeed, as the introductory chapter to this book cautions us, there can be no universalising narrative of the pandemic. And evidently, the conversation at the badminton club could only have been spoken from privileged social locations in the global north boasting a well-functioning public health system and a robust social infrastructure. As is by now tragically well known, the Indian experience with COVID-19 is dramatically and devastatingly different and, as this book powerfully brings out, the easy-going air of slight bewilderment at having come through almost unscathed that defined the small talk in Oslo is entirely absent from most Indian conversations about COVID-19. As Rahul Ranjan shows in his introduction, Indian conversations about COVID-19 continue to gravitate not around its "strangeness" but around grief, loss, mourning, and pain. And throughout the book, we are reminded of how shock and trauma still define India's pandemic experience: "the virus", Rahul writes, "runs deep as a trope of trauma and grief in the everyday lives of Indians now".

The trauma and grief that so persistently live on, however, are largely attributable to political rather than virological and biological processes, a point that is reiterated across chapters. True to his autocratic style of governance, Prime Minister Modi announced India's first lockdown on March 23, 2020, without any prior warning, giving citizens a mere four hours to prepare. Those who could stock up on basic necessities and retreated to their homes where they could minimise viral exposure by settling into new temporal and spatial routines centred on working from home and ordering necessities online through delivery services. Those who could not—the poor, the slum dwellers, the working classes, the labour migrants, small traders, and petty commodity producers of all kinds—were left to fend almost entirely for themselves. Migrant workers, in particular, many stranded hundreds or sometimes thousands of kilometres away from home, were shamefully victimised in a dual sense: The government abdicated all responsibility for their welfare, leaving hundreds of thousands, if not millions, of migrant workers with no other option than to return to their native villages or towns through whatever means available, crisscrossing the country on foot or bicycle in search of helping hands and social support. Yet while doing so, many became—as Manjesh Rana's chapter shows—victims of violent police excesses as they were shamed, humiliated, and beaten up for violating the rules of the lockdown. As elsewhere, the distribution of suffering and pain in a pandemic context was highly uneven, fractured systematically through the prism of class as well as caste and gender.

The rationale of a lockdown is not only to minimise viral exposure and spread; it is also crucially about buying time to boost public health systems and to sufficiently equip the various parts of this system—materially, infrastructurally, psychologically, and logistically—to deal with what is in store. In India, this was never going to be an easy task, given the country's woefully inadequate and systematically under-prioritised public health sector, which has been neglected by shifting central and state governments for decades. Still, one might have anticipated that a popularly elected government would do its utmost to ramp up the public health sector as a matter of urgent priority and as effectively as possible despite all economic constraints and sedimented historical legacies of neglect. But this is not what happened in India. As several studies—both academic and journalistic—have documented, the Modi government's response during the extended lockdown was overwhelmingly one of inaction. This meant that when the second pandemic "wave" hit India in the spring of 2021, the impact was devastating. For weeks on end, thousands of people succumbed to the pandemic every day, with hundreds of thousands of new cases officially registered daily. The actual figure was undoubtedly much higher, and the pandemic hardly left anyone untouched; all my Indian friends and colleagues who I was in touch with at the time had a relative, a friend, a colleague, or a neighbour who fell gravely ill, leading near and dear ones to embark on a desperate search for oxygen, a hospital bed, and medical care, all of which were in all too short supply. Rahul Ranjan invokes Alf Nilsen's work on the pandemic to mount a critique of the Modi regime's authoritarian populist mishandling of the pandemic, but to me, the crucial operative term in Nilsen's work is "social murder". The concept comes from Friedrich Engels, who, in his study of the working poor in 19th-century England, used it to capture how the working class in an industrialising society lived under conditions in which they could neither retain health nor live long. "The perverse workings" of political-economic structures, in other words (and these are Nilsen's words), preyed "on the working poor through social murder". To Nilsen, something very similar unfolded in India during the pandemic when the Modi regime not only failed to rein in and ameliorate the workings of social murder but actively sought to further the consolidation of the very power relations that produced these workings in the first place.

This book courageously and meticulously brings out how the debris of an epochal pandemic crisis now lies scattered all around us. In the social life of communities, kin, and neighbourhoods; in the grief and mourning of individuals and families struggling to heal; and in the long-term insurmountable suffering inflicted on marginalised communities in particular. The book admirably lives up to its promise to document varied pandemic experiences as a stepping stone towards formulating new theoretical frameworks and more transparent decision-making processes. But just as importantly, the experiences and narratives presented throughout the book also, in their own right, contain a moral force grounded in lived experience on which to build a broader and perhaps more foundational critique of the operations of power and the highly unequal distribution of suffering and risk in contemporary India.

Kenneth Bo Nielsen
Oslo, June 7, 2024

Introduction

Rahul Ranjan

> *"Our mourning, our letting grieve over the loss of loved ones is an expression of our commitment a form of communication and communion".*
>
> (hooks 2000)

Grief fills our lives today. Every loss, especially when we fail to hold a last bodily departure, leaves in us a deep void. Mourning, as hooks said, shows us the ultimate expression of that loss when rendered visible. Through the treacherous, often fraught with immense pain, those departed form a "continuing bond" with us (Millar and Lopez-Cantero 2022). Mourning forms the basis for making our loss a generative force—unifying the loose ends of differences into a shared sense of belonging. Historically, epochal crises have inaugurated new arrays of thinking. The pandemic, a crisis of unprecedented scale and impact, also leads us through another opportunity to reconcile vast differences that shape our lives and loss. Roy has famously opined that the pandemic is a "portal" that describes the insufferable bearing of inequality on our shoulders and how we may either carry the carcass of past mistakes or imagine a better future (Roy 2020). Furthermore, she claims that "the tragedy is immediate, real, epic and unfolding before our eyes. But it isn't new. It is the wreckage of a train that has been careening down the track for years."

As the shock of the pandemic brought the world to a standstill, people began to think more acutely about the importance of solidarity and the lack of political strength. The shared sense of loss permeated the borders in the restricted capacity to move freely. In this stillness, the "we" emerged more strongly. In his compelling book, "Bodies on the Barricade," Prakash develops a rich milieu of how bodily suffering expands our imagination of crisis—illustrating the limits of freedom. He writes, "The shared space and feeling of breathlessness and yearning can offer the possibility of common ground where all these differences might meet and engage one another. In the loss of ideas and enthusiasm, the 'we' becomes our last hope, a witness of our last struggle" (Prakash 2023, 28).

This sense of loss, as eloquently expressed by Prakash, also drew poets, writers, and imaginative practitioners to respond (Prakash 2023). Such responses filled a gaping hole people felt locked in their homes, while others,

DOI: 10.4324/9781003591641-1

such as migrants in India, were forced to walk back home. The pandemic is not a flattening inequality crisis but rather a moment of its pronouncement. It was a visceral display of unequal forces of material that structure our lives. Sandro Mazzedra drew our attention to the fragility of the system in his work by calling for "care of the common" (Mezzadra 2020). Each in their home—hiding away from the fear of contagion—also bore witness to those who could not hide but be exposed, driven out or, as Prakash asks (about migrants): "Where will they move now? Perhaps they will move to another site, to another city, to another job in other capacities . . . they will be back in the city again, as outsiders, to keep the city moving" (Prakash 2023, 96). Assembling care for any reparative world requires labour. Racial minorities, healthcare workers, women, and other labouring classes became shields to the public as frontline care providers (Mezzadra 2020). Many of them lost their lives. The crisis, therefore, entrenched the long-standing wedging gap in society—exposing the weakened public infrastructure.

Many have argued that the pandemic revealed structural fault lines that are decisive in managing any crisis. These fault lines feature through caste, indigeneity, class and gender in India—forming an assemblage of differences that structure access to public infrastructure. Samaddar, in his compelling on COVID crisis in India, argues that the "pandemic lays bare the extent to which individual health depends on the health of everyone in the community, while public healthcare has been eroded through decades of austerity policies, privatization, and inadequate planning" (Samaddar 2020, 16). The gradual withdrawal of funding from the public infrastructure enforced high "demands on government institutions' capacity, and especially on local government institutions that are comparatively weak in the global south" (Levine et al. 2023). These also manifested at the macro level through stagnation in the economic growth that disproportionately disadvantages the marginalised communities. Reports note that since 2022, "the structure of the workforce is skewed more towards self-employment than it was before the slowdown, and earnings remain depressed. The impact was strongly gendered with women being more affected" (State of Working India 2023: Social Identities and Labour Market Outcomes 2023). These factors contributed to the making of an epochal crisis.

Pandemic, an Epochal Crisis

COVID-19 has introduced a new scale of crisis across the world. Origins in zoonotic viral composition, COVID-19 has exposed the systemic weakness in governing the populous—causing an emergent and expansive crisis. Traces of disruption that emerged from the virus as transmittable to bodies, of course, were not limited to it. As Hale noted,

> COVID-19 attacks the human body, but it is largely the body politic that defends us against it. While we wait for vaccines and treatments,

> we depend on health systems, governments, and the actions of others to detect the virus, control its spread, and break the chain of infection in the public health sectors, social welfare system and food security
> (2020)

In other words, the virus becomes a metaphor to expose both the capacity and fragility of a system constituted by political institutions, actors, and modes of governance. These varied units interact in complex ways to provide a framework for governance to mitigate a crisis.

A core feature of any crisis rests in urgency: the urgency to respond, tackle and mitigate. While the virus outbreak is hugely damaging, as we have learned, it also causes a long-term impact on our bodies. Sellnow and Seeger define the crisis as "a specific, unexpected, non-routine event or series of events that create high uncertainty" (Sellnow and Seeger 2013, 7). Aggravated uncertainties triggered by systemic failures often incapacitate the institutions in responding to the urgency. The inability to control the spread and prepare a more comprehensive strategy heightens the crisis. COVID has ongoing effects on bodies and the system (Bambra et al. 2021). It is a multiscale crisis that creates fissures in political processes—often granting extraordinary power to the state. This makes politics a key tool in structuring the crisis. Lipscy argues that "the politics of Covid 19 is the politics of crisis" because it "compels leaders to make high-stakes decisions under conditions of threat, uncertainty, and time pressure" (2020, 99).

Furthermore, a crisis, whether COVID or others, often emerges as a "situation that threatens significant harm to a country's populations or basic values and compels a political response under time pressure and uncertainty" (Lipscy 2020, 100). In this way, a crisis can present new opportunities to reimagine political institutions or entrench the existing problems. A crisis such as COVID not only poses a significant threat to economic activities by holding hostage the circular flow of trade but also weakens the internal policies that govern micro-scale businesses dependent on mobility (Sumner et al. 2020). Political processes that provide support in such a situation are confronted with a problem that is not evident and originated outside the virus. Therefore, the response by political parties is crucial to ensuring preparedness for mitigating the effect. However, as Lipscy rightly points out, "Covid response came to be seen broadly in terms of national success or failure. . . . In short, the politics of Covid-19 is best understood as the politics of crisis" (Lipscy 2020, 105).

Besides the administrative disruption and political instability, a crisis also leaves a deep imprint on the social life of communities. They often manifest in terms of long-lasting trauma that emerges from the loss—creating personal and social cohesion fissures. While it may seem that the world has gradually returned to normalcy, the lingering grief of those who survived the loss often stays. Control of mobility through stringent lockdown meant less, and, in some cases, none of the family members could perform the last rites of passage. Funerary rituals constitute the social life of an individual. By virtue of being human, it is bestowed upon us.

Denial of accessing that last passage could also be, as Richardson et al. wrote, "furthermore, distressing 'unfinished businesses with the dead—more likely when we cannot say goodbye—might lead to unusually prolonged or complicated grief" (Richardson et al. 2021, 90). A crisis story, hence, is multifaceted and often involves complicated relationships between institutions, individuals and communities. With the timely interventions made by large-scale inoculation of vaccines, even though unequal in distribution and, in the worst case, controlled by the global north, the world achieved some stability. However, there is a need for a comprehensive study that helps situate a place-based and case-specific analysis of the COVID crisis. Even though a pandemic, by definition, is a global crisis, the existing inequality deepens the effects differently.

Burgeoning literature shows how the impacts of this crisis are interspersed with various issues, including migration, mortality, poverty, illness, and economic instability, amongst others (Sharma et al. 2021). Therefore, this volume intends to escape any universalising narrative of suffering and provide specific strands of inequality that shape the lives of those at the margins of power. Specifically, in countries such as India, where social realities are not always exclusively determined by class but also significantly by caste, gender, and religion, it is crucial to document varied experiences. These experiences enrich our understanding of a pandemic by providing insights into a complex web of relationships between society, state, and institutions. In doing so, this volume examines the political, economic, and social impacts of COVID-19 on the marginalised communities in India and the ways in which it was further entrenched. To situate the *crisis* in India as the context for the study, the section below provides an introduction and critical contributions to the volume.

COVID: An Indian Story

On April 18, 2021, I landed in Oslo from New Delhi. As I was given a separate passage to test for COVID and then escorted in a bus to a hotel for 10 days quarantine, streets in India abound with heaps of deceased bodies. Everyone on that flight was a suspect in the virus. While I received emails informing the removal of all restrictions and a majority population reaching the end of double inoculation of vaccines in Norway, India reported more than five million cases of COVID-19 (The Lancet 2021). I was profoundly inarticulate to express this seething grief that grew inside as I witnessed the horrific visuals on screen. With no space to perform the last rites of loved ones, Indians turned parking space into a makeshift cemetery ground. Every morsel of food in Oslo's airport hotel seemed like a heavy lump of survivor's guilt for the next 10 days.

As bodies began to float in the river and numbers soared in this second wave of COVID in India, I anticipated a distressed call from my ageing parents in India. Escaping the cruelty of time, the *wave*—a word often used to invoke poetic rendition of seashore was squishing the last breath of those struggling to breathe—seemed impossible. Social media was saturated with requests for oxygen and hospitals, while phones from friends and families buzzed endlessly seeking help. This virtual collective within and outside India exhausted their resources and will to fetch breath—literally oxygen for friends, families, and acquaintances as bodies mound outside hospitals. While in Norway, people geared up for the Constitution Day celebration after the end of the lockdown, Indians assembled strength to survive this epochal disaster. I use this anecdote as a cursory description to magnify the contradiction and irony of what constitutes a pandemic, which is assumed to hold universal urgency and crisis but often exposes stark, unequal realities of the world.

This crisis has further entrenched the existing inequalities across India's social, economic, and political spectrum. Various factors contributed to the colossal loss. Foremost, this is the lack of coordinated governance that coincided with the lack of communication, which is "embedded social norms to create a sense of public awareness and political will to awaken the public to the crisis" (Dutta and Fischer 2021). As it seemed in the early period, a viral outbreak quickly descended into an unrelenting "social suffering" caused by the lockdown and abysmal poverty (Nilsen 2022). Many of these coincided with the lack thereof and mismanagement of vaccines that should have been "equitable to access as a human right" (Sirohi 2021).

While the register of political and administrative failure is apparent, the virus runs deep as a trope of trauma and grief in the everyday lives of Indians now. Far from being transient and invisible, the emotional cost of the pandemic is enormous—transforming the lives of marginalised communities. Deep traumatic experiences shaped everyday social conduct and ritual performance. From ghats to the crematorium, this virus changed the "imaginative possibilities of grieving the loss" (Ranjan 2021). In this passage, ordinary people defeated by the state, grounded their faith in closed kinship networks, neighbours, and, unsurprisingly, social media networking—assembling resources needed to save their loved ones. However, the popular representation of COVID—especially within media, was driven an immediacy to report on the tragedy as the consequence of the virus, leaving little or no scope for highlighting what I argue as the "structural indifference to inequality". The scale of the viral outbreak in rural India and underreporting brought minimal admission to the grim reality that continues to shape people's lives (Koshy 2021). This was a crisis India had not anticipated or wilfully ignored. To be able to tell this story, let me revert to March 2020 and provide a sequential chain of tragedy.

In December 2019, when COVID was beginning to emerge as a news item in the international media without sufficient attention to its grave arrival, the streets of India were claimed by protestors challenging the controversial Citizenship Amendment Act (CAA). An Act that proposed to disenfranchise, specifically Muslims, through a complex web of bureaucracy, evidence, and proof—jeopardising the core secular commitment (Nielsen and Nilsen 2021). An immediate response to this move (CAA) led to an intensified protest sprawling nationwide. These protests displayed powerful demonstrations of claims and the practice of democratic dissent. However, the transmission of the virus also began to intensify by late January 2020. Little did we know about a pandemic on the horizon; Indian authority remained uncertain until early March. While various circulars were issued to impose conservative restrictions on the municipal level, India awaited a nationwide lockdown.

Chronicling the Event and Argument of the Volume

On March 23, 2020, the Prime Minister of India, Narendra Modi, the leader of the Bharatiya Janata Party, the Hindu right-wing, announced a nationwide lockdown. Known for making dramatic appearances to announce the news that often has had large-scale impacts, such as demonetisation, Modi ushered the nation with his speech into a huge lockdown. Bringing the whole country to a standstill, the Indian story of COVID began to sprawl through different narratives. Perhaps, as some studies show, the first wave of COVID in 2020, where "the original strain of the virus was 'less fit', hence could not penetrate the strong natural immunity barrier supposedly present in most Indian hosts. This barrier could have been in the form of cross-protection due to expo sure to other coronaviruses" (Chinnaswamy 2021, 2). Even as the strain was mild and casualties were relatively lower in the first wave, the lockdown wreaked havoc on many who live on the cracks of Indian society. As Roy noted, these cracks are also places within cities—in other words, there is a city where state institutions and economic activities are conducted and a non-city (cracks) where poor, dispossessed, and migrants live.

In this brief introduction to the volume, I explain two specific points that highlight the COVID crisis in India. Firstly, India's population of 1.3 billion was given four hours short notice during the first wave, which either left a huge migrant population stranded or forced them to on foot walk back home. In subsequent weeks following this exodus, the government released a package to provide help but did not include circular migrants. Secondly, the second wave of COVID exposed a combination of weak medical infrastructure and the need for more political leadership. Considering these two strands as paradigmatic because of the scale of their implication, India set out towards a long struggle.

As this volume shows, I argue that COVID revealed an entangled crisis—exemplifying weak structures of governance, lack of political leadership, and primarily India's underdeveloped public health infrastructure that receives a fraction of the economy (Ghosh 2020). Specifically, the crisis caused long-term impairment of disadvantaged groups through structural inaccessibility to medical infrastructure, and, in other circumstances, they were subject to excessive use of power by a state official (chapter by Manjesh). The crisis is entangled because it distributes insurmountable suffering in the long term to those who are faced with structural disadvantages. The vulnerabilities are constituted by various strands of the precarious labour market in India. This includes a long-standing sub-contractual nature as the core of the migrant flow from various states (Bihar, Jharkhand, Odisha, and Bengal)—allowing them to be hired cheaply and unregulated by any enforceable contract that protects their interest (Pattenden 2016; Srivastava and Sutradhar 2016). The *internal alienness* of the labour force defined by their location and precarity was further deepened by the existing federal fiscal deficit (Shah and Lerche 2020). It systematically limits their capacity to either attend to or provide the required support to reduce the crisis's scale. Ironically, the states of Bihar, Jharkhand, and Odisha, which consist of the highest net out-migration of labourers, also invariably are fiscally deficient or have a reduced capacity to provide degrees of safety. Therefore, the migrants who serve as the backbone of the "India shining" story began to walk barefoot home and start populating the screen display of Indian television—displaying the state's collective moral and political failure. Srivastava shows how "[t]he exodus of the migrants began in the first week of lockdown, but the severe governmental response pushed them back to their shelters, or they interned in government shelters. However, there was no way to contain these migrant workers once there was news of an extension of the lockdown. Millions of workers, often accompanied by their family members, including young children began walking back to their villages—often thousands of miles away" (Srivastava 2020, 873). As internally differentiated groups, migrants, including Dalits, Adivasi, and the working class, while walking for days in scorching heat and without much food, lost their lives. Upon seeking a request on the same, the Ministry of Labour and Employment, through a written reply said, "no such data is available" (Web Desk 2020).

In his recent scholarship, Nilsen has argued that India's lockdown can be understood in "terms of how the lockdown served as a form of spectacle, intended to project a public image of Modi as a strongman leader capable of swift action to defend Indian citizens against the pandemic, and argue that this has to be understood in terms of the political logic of Modi's authoritarian populism" (Nilsen 2022, 2). This analysis combines the ongoing rise of right-wing politics in India with the pandemic—presenting the politics of COVID-19 as the politics of crisis. Nilsen shows how Modi used the crisis as a form of spectacle to "defy the law of political gravity" and, in fact, improved his approval rating during the lockdown (Nilsen 2022, 5). Others have characterised COVID-19 in India as a systematic failure of the government and its inability to constitute a nationwide policy. Roy writes, "This virus is an international problem. To deal with it, decision-making, at least on the control and administration of the pandemic, will need to pass into the hands of some sort of non-partisan body consisting of members of the ruling party, members of the opposition, and health and public policy experts" (Roy 2021). The national coordination and impartial data availability help assess pandemic and potential risk more robustly. Unfortunately, the lack of data and unpreparedness of political will aggravated the nature of the crisis in India. This was acutely combined with inadequate support measures ("21 Days and Counting: Covid-19 Lockdown, Migrant Workers, and the Inadequacy of Welfare Measures in India" 2020). The central government delegated these measures that clearly undermined the scale of impact and reliance on migrants. These failures were marked by heterogeneous factors contributing to a massive failure of both virus contamination and wide-scale distress faced by migrants.

Amongst others, the lack of coordination between states and, more generally, the social protections severely impacted the migrants (Abraham et al. 2022). As a huge proportion of the economy relies on the "informal economy," social protection becomes the most crucial tool for protection in case of any catastrophe. These social protections suffer a massive blow due to the unequal development pattern with a wave of labour migration to urban centres. Urban centres have a huge concentration of labour in the hinterlands. The flow of circular migration sustains the informality, which is generative of both profit and absolute surplus from labour (Jan 2013).

Often sustained by close-knit social and kinship networks, the circular migration abounds the Indian labour market. It provides a casualised labour force at the highest minimum wage rate, thereby removing the contractual obligation towards safety and various protectionary measures. This perpetuates the maintenance of both low-economic requirements for extended labour support and the sustaining caste primacy that defines it (Kundu and Sarangi 2007). Such hierarchised socially differentiated repertoire provides for and enables condition to sustain the circular migration. These patterns often involve precarious networks of people drawn out of agrarian distress in rural areas or socially excluded classes with limited resources. During COVID-19, when the social buffer was fragmented and informality ceased to exist, the fractures in the labour precarity became glaringly evident despite government support.

COVID-19, as a moment of crisis, also explicates contradictions and its entangled relations with capitalism and its counterparts in Indian society. Surbhi et al., in their well-grounded and extended research, argue that "[t]he economic reproduction of the non-capitalist household enterprises may be sustained even by compressing consumption levels in the absence of alternative livelihood opportunities, especially during times of economic crisis. These dynamics allow the enterprises to act as a sink for the surplus population, as evinced by the expansion of non-capitalist self-employment globally and the worsening situation of the informal working population observed during the COVID-19 pandemic" (Kesar et al. 2022). These contradictions, in turn, deepen the entangled crisis—ceasing the growth at the bottom, where fissures of COVID effects are prominent. Effectively, such patterns of permanent labour circulation within informal and exploitative forms also influenced post-COVID recovery. In his work, Manish shows how recovery is crucially impacted by the long-term impairment of labour exploitation (Maskara 2023).

Therefore, this volume consolidates and makes a cutting-edge contribution to revealing different strands of entanglement, which enabled the crisis to permeate into social and political life during COVID-19 in India. Through grounded, empirically rich, and theoretically sharp undertakings, the volume features key dynamics of governance that crucially shaped the management of COVID-19. The analysis throughout the volume deepens how COVID-19 as an epochal crisis in India highlights the nature and scope of medical emergencies that could lead to systemic disruptions—furthering inequalities regardless of a sector-specific nature. The volume promises to display clarity on how and why specific communities, including migrants, artists, nomadic, and especially Adivasi (Indigenous peoples) who bore persistent inequalities before COVID were further entrenched into fragmented structures of support. As this volume shows, many perilous consequences should be considered as a long-term reconstruction of policy design that could accommodate not only emergency measures but also reparative steps in ensuring that structural inequalities are reduced and strong safeguards are provided.

Structure and Contributions of the Volume

Any crisis, therefore, requires comprehensive understanding and timely intervention. A pandemic is a portal, as Roy pointed out. It allows us to reassess the idea of risk and how political decisions play a significant role in addressing any crisis. COVID is not limited to the viral outbreak but is also related to the emergent climate crisis and how it deepens the existing inequality in society (Castree et al. 2014). Social scientists are crucial in offering critical insights into knowledge that can be effectively applied to normative judgement, policy, and broader societal inquiries. An essential contribution in this direction is to advance the understanding of the COVID crisis in India by providing empirical evidence and widening the discussion of the theoretical framework.

The volume structure is organised thematically to respond to the idea of crisis. The contributions in the volume combine robust accounts of narratives, social inequality, empirically informed policy analysis, grievances, and political processes that shaped the structure of governance and resilience during the COVID-19 pandemic. The reason for thematic inquiry emerges from the geographical diversity of case studies arising from specific socio-political and economic processes and the complex interactions between institutions and governance. While a few contributions, such as Manjesh Rana, Aashish Xaxa, and Afreen Gani Faridi, evaluate deeply enmeshed power relations between institutions and policies at both national and regional levels, other contributors, including Sushmita and Rashmi Kumari, provide ethnographic details and micro-level analysis of broader long-standing challenges faced by the marginalised communities at the margins of the nation. Aparna Agarwal, Rituparna Patgiri, and Pratik Mishra bring to the fore the deeply complicated nature of the "workforce" co-constituted by caste and class. They demonstrate how the ideas of labour, whether part of the creative industries (mobile theatre), manual labour work (brick kilns), or those who worked as "frontline," were confronted with precarity coupled with the existing disadvantage. Finally, Nishant Sirohi and Ritwika Patgiri showcase flaws in the resilience and recovery policy design. In some cases, it is the lack thereof of a comprehensive vaccine policy, whereas in others, it is the understanding of the intersectional scope of climate change and COVID-19. Both chapters build or suggest a comprehensive overview for creating pathways to mitigate the crisis.

All the contributions in the volume present empirically rich and detailed governance accounts that were decisive in shaping the policy during the COVID-19 pandemic. I outline their key arguments and questions hereafter. Sushmita's chapter on "The task before rebuilding: COVID-19 in Jharkhand, impact, and responses" assesses the government's response during COVID-19 to demonstrate the impact of COVID-19 on Adivasis and forest-dwelling people, especially during the second wave. Their chapter traces various media reports, government websites, and other advisories to see the state's response. The chapter builds pathways towards envisioning good governance by drawing on different anecdotal and narrative evidence from civil society actors and community members. Similarly, Rashmi Kumari, in her chapter "Navigating Medical Neglect and Care: COVID-19 Management and Adivasi Societies," explores the fear of vaccination among the rural Adivasi population of Chhattisgarh is rooted in historical encounters between the "modern" health systems and the Adivasi communities. The chapter argues that the COVID-19 crisis was one of many crises the Adivasi community has faced over the last century and that their suspicion towards vaccinations cannot be brushed under the popular perceptions of Adivasi being ignorant, superstitious, and innocent village folks. Instead, Adivasi communities' reluctance should be understood along with the historical, political, and medical negligence of the Adivasi communities by the governing systems.

Grounded in the large survey and in-depth interviews, the chapter "Policing the Pandemic" by Manjesh Rana renders the key tenets of governance and excessive use of power visible. The chapter is motivated to understand the facets of policing in India during the pandemic by looking at the citizen–police interactions during the lockdown, the handling of the crisis, and the emergence of new challenges for the law enforcement apparatus. The chapter presents how police often resorted to the practice of humiliating and shaming the "violators," with the socio-economically disadvantaged section, including migrant workers, disproportionally bearing the burden of such police excesses, pushing them further to the margins. Similarly, Aashish

Xaxa, in his chapter "Covid-19 and the Indigenous migrants' Question in Urban India," engages and addresses the problems of tribal migrant workers from two different geographical regions of the country—Central India and the Northeast. The chapter illustrates how Indian cities are built on the hard labour and exploitation of migrant workers, but they remain indifferent to the consciousness of the architects, planners, corporations, and middle class, and they are often considered part of the problem in cities. Afreen Gani Faridi, in his chapter "Intersections of Covid-19 within Nomadic Lives," examines the Gujjar-Bakarwal tribe of Jammu and Kashmir—one of the largest tribal groups which traverse across the Himalayas along with their flock. The chapter analyses environmental and extractive governmentality during the COVID-19 pandemic in actuating dispossession and sedentarisation through the criminalisation of a community—to catalyse a shift away from their transhumant natures.

By interweaving the livelihood, frontline work, and labour mobility, Pratik Mishra traces the period of disruption from COVID as a continuation of suspension and precarity imposed within brick kiln workers' lives. This chapter presents how the public health concerns of COVID were negotiated within a context where kiln workers remain unable to afford or access formal or qualified healthcare, save for a few life occasions. This exclusion makes it unlikely that a scientific discourse on the virus will filter through to replace traditional modalities of understanding disease and contagion. Such interaction between the deeply embedded relationships between identities and inequalities is not uncommon in India. For instance, in her chapter "The Last of Frontline Workers," Aparna Agarwal explores the intricate connection between COVID-19 and the state of sanitation workers and waste workers in Delhi. The chapter argues that even though the pandemic has brought issues of public health to the forefront, the issues surrounding sanitation and waste work are still predominantly shaped by caste hierarchies and practices of stigmatisation. At the same time, Rituparna Patgiri's chapter traces the impact on the creative industry constituted by the non-organised labour force. It showcases how the mobile theatre, a significant source of employment in rural Assam in the pre-pandemic years, faced enormous challenges due to the disruption of performance. The chapter argues that the brunt of the adverse consequences of the pandemic borne by the technical artists and other workers, most of whom belong to the lower caste and class, is not just economical but has also influenced the cultural practice of mobile theatre.

In his chapter "Right to Health and India's Covid-19 Vaccine Policy," Nishant Sirohi maps out the challenges in India's COVID-19 vaccine policy, which failed to ensure adequate availability and access to vaccines. The chapter argues that even though socio-economic rights are not justiciable under the Indian Constitution, the courts over the years have evolved a jurisprudence that presents a framework to enforce the right to health in India. However, in framing the COVID-19 vaccine policy, the government has failed to consider the directives of the courts related to access to healthcare, treatment, and essential medicines. Finally, the chapter "Community Resilience in the Western Himalayas: Lessons from the Pandemic" by Ritwika Patgiri demonstrates how the Himalayan states, which saw depopulation and the emergence of ghost villages before the pandemic, witnessed a trend of reverse migration. By centring on community resilience, the chapter tries to understand how the COVID-19 pandemic has affected the lives of people in a region battling climate change, water crisis, and natural disasters during the pandemic and how the communities have responded to these challenges.

Conclusion

This volume comprises comprehensive contributions from social scientists, humanities scholars and independent researchers spanning various disciplines, some actively involved in frontline relief efforts (Hulme et al. 2020). The aim is to build a diverse body of knowledge to facilitate more transparent understanding of the decision-making processes and "dismantle unhelpful hierarchies of knowledge" (Hulme et al. 2020, 1). The contributors emphasise how the COVID crisis is deeply intertwined with unequal power dynamics, governance issues, and longstanding social inequalities in India. The concept of crisis serves as a framework for understanding COVID management and as a political space that brings attention to long-standing unresolved problems such as migration, inadequate public health infrastructure, and social disparities.

This volume advocates for more thorough studies that can help understand the long-term effects of viral outbreaks on human health and the environment by promoting an intersectional analysis of the COVID crisis. It aims to contribute to political science, public health, anthropology, sociology, and public policy studies by addressing livelihood, migration, policing, vaccines, and community resilience. As the virus evolves and the crisis persists, the publication envisions further research to develop comprehensive frameworks for understanding and addressing these challenges. Finally, the contributions in this publication enhance our understanding of crisis management and underscore the need for inclusive, fair, and well-informed policy interventions. Integrating interdisciplinary perspectives, focusing on the experiences of marginalised communities, and highlighting the role of governance offers valuable insights and lessons for addressing future crises.

References

21 days and counting: Covid-19 lockdown, migrant workers, and the inadequacy of welfare measures in India. 2020. Accessed 20 May 2024. https://ruralindiaonline.org/en/library/resource/21-days-and-counting-covid-19-lockdown-migrant-workers-and-the-inadequacy-of-welfare-measures-in-india/.

Abraham, R., Basole, A. and Kesar, S. 2022. Down and out? The gendered impact of the covid-19 pandemic on India's labour market. *Economia Politica* 39 (1): 101–28. https://doi.org/10.1007/s40888-021-00234-8.

Bambra, C., Lynch, J. and Smith, K. E. 2021. *The Unequal Pandemic*. Policy Press. https://doi.org/10.51952/9781447361251.

Castree, N., Adams, W. M., Barry, J., Brockington, D., Büscher, B., Corbera, E., Demeritt, D., Duffy, R., Felt, E., Neves, K., Newell, P., Pellizzoni, L., Rigby, K., Robbins, P., Robin, L., Rose, D. B., Ross, A., Schlosberg, D., Sörlin, S., West, P., Whitehead, M. and Wynn, B. 2014. Changing the intellectual climate. *Nature Climate Change* 4 (9): 763–68. https://doi.org/10.1038/nclimate2339.

Chinnaswamy, S. 2021. Understanding the devastating second wave of Covid-19 pandemic in India. *American Journal of Human Biology* 33 (6). https://doi.org/10.1002/ajhb.23671.

Dutta, A. and Fischer, H. W. 2021. The local governance of Covid-19: Disease prevention and social security in rural India. *World Development* 138 (February): 105234. https://doi.org/10.1016/j.worlddev.2020.105234.

Ghosh, J. 2020. "A critique of the Indian government's response to the Covid-19 pandemic." *Journal of Industrial and Business Economics* 47 (3): 519–30. https://doi.org/10.1007/s40812-020-00170-x.

Hale, T. 2020. An immune system for the body politic: Using social science to control Covid-19. In *Voices*. University of Oxford.

Hooks, B. 2000. *All About Love*. New York: Haper Collins.

Hulme, M., Lidskog, R., White, J. M. and Standring, A. 2020. Social scientific knowledge in times of crisis: What climate change can learn from coronavirus (and vice versa). *WIREs Climate Change* 11 (4). https://doi.org/10.1002/wcc.656.

Jan, B. 2013. *At Work in the Informal Economy of India: A Perspective from the Bottom Up*. Delhi: Oxford University Press.

Kesar, S., Bhattacharya, S. and Banerjee, L. 2022. Contradictions and crisis in the world of work: Informality, precarity and the pandemic. *Development and Change* 53 (6): 1254–82. https://doi.org/10.1111/dech.12733.

Koshy, J. 2021. Are states under-reporting Covid-19 cases? *The Hindu*, August.

Kundu, A. and Sarangi, N. 2007. Migration, employment status and poverty: An analysis across urban centres. *Economic and Political Weekly* 42 (4): 299–306.

The Lancet. 2021. India's Covid-19 emergency. *The Lancet* 397 (10286): 1683. https://doi.org/10.1016/S0140-6736(21)01052-7.

Levine, A. C., Park, A., Adhikari, A., Alejandria, M. C. P., Bradlow, B. H., Lopez-Portillo, M. F., Mutwafy, S., Zumbyte, I. and Heller, P. 2023. The role of Civil Society Organizations (CSOs) in the Covid-19 response across the global South: A multinational, qualitative study. *PLOS Global Public Health* 3 (9): e0002341. https://doi.org/10.1371/journal.pgph.0002341.

Lipscy, P. Y. 2020. Covid-19 and the politics of crisis. *International Organization* 74 (S1): E98–E127. https://doi.org/10.1017/S0020818320000375.

Maskara, M. 2023. Reproducing precariousness of labour: Post-lockdown reorganisation of labour in building construction in India. In Dutta, R. (ed.) *Pandemic and Precarity*. Kolkata: Sampark, 144167.

Mezzadra, S. 2020. Politics of struggles in the time of pandemic. *Verso*, 17 March. https://www.versobooks.com/en-gb/blogs/news/4598-politics-of-struggles-in-the-time-of-pandemic.

Millar, B. and Lopez-Cantero, P. 2022. Grief, continuing bonds, and unreciprocated love. *Southern Journal of Philosophy* 60 (3): 413–36. https://doi.org/10.1111/sjp.12462.

Nielsen, K. B. and Nilsen, A. G. 2021. Hindu nationalist statecraft and Modi's authoritarian populism. In Widmalm, S. (ed.) *Routledge Handbook of Autocratization in South Asia*. London: Routledge, 92–100. https://doi.org/10.4324/9781003042211.

Nilsen, A. G. 2022. India's pandemic: Spectacle, social murder and authoritarian politics in a lockdown nation. *Globalizations* 19 (3): 466–86. https://doi.org/10.1080/14747731.2021.1935019.

Pattenden, J. 2016. Working at the margins of global production networks: Local labour control regimes and rural-based labourers in South India. *Third World Quarterly* 37 (10): 1809–33. https://doi.org/10.1080/01436597.2016.1191939.

Prakash, B. 2023. Body on the barricades: Life, art and resistance. In *Contemporary India*. Delhi: LeftWord.

Ranjan, R. 2021. Mourning on the ghat: Bagmati, a short note. *Doing Sociology*, 15 May.

Richardson, L., Ratcliffe, M., Millar, B. and Byrne, E. 2021. The Covid-19 pandemic and the bounds of grief. *Think* 20 (57): 89–101. https://doi.org/10.1017/S1477175620000366.

Roy, A. 2020. *The Pandemic Is a Portal*. https://www.ft.com/content/10d8f5e8-74eb-11ea-95fe-fcd274e920ca.

Roy, A. 2021. It's Not Enough to Say the Govt Has Failed. We Are Witnessing a Crime Against Humanity. *The Wire*, 29 April 2021. https://thewire.in/government/india-covid-19-government-crime-against-humanity.

Samaddar, R. 2020. *Borders of an Epidemic: Covid-19 and Migrant Workers*. Calcutta: Mahanirban.

Sellnow, T. L. and Seeger, M. W. 2013. *Theorizing Crisis Communication*. Wiley-Blackwell.

Shah, A. and Lerche, J. 2020. Migration and the invisible economies of care: Production, social reproduction and seasonal migrant labour in India. *Transactions of the Institute of British Geographers* 45 (4): 719–34. https://doi.org/10.1111/tran.12401.

Sharma, J. R., Sharma, A. and Kapilashrami, A. 2021. Covid-19 and the precarity of low-income migrant workers in Indian cities. *Society and Culture in South Asia* 7 (1): 48–62. https://doi.org/10.1177/2393861720975618.

Sirohi, N. 2021. Right to equitable access to Covid-19 vaccination—if not now, then when? *Observer Research Foundation*, April 9.

Srivastava, R. 2020. Labour migration, vulnerability, and development policy: The pandemic as inflexion point? *The Indian Journal of Labour Economics* 63 (4): 859–83. https://doi.org/10.1007/s41027-020-00301-x.

Srivastava, R. and Sutradhar, R. 2016. Labour migration to the construction sector in India and its impact on rural poverty. *Indian Journal of Human Development* 10 (1): 27–48. https://doi.org/10.1177/0973703016648028.

State of Working India 2023: Social Identities and Labour Market Outcomes. Bengaluru: Centre for Sustainable Employment, Azim Premji University. Accessed 5 July 2024. https://azimpremjiuniversity.edu.in/publications/2023/report/state-of-working-india-2023-social-identities-and-labour-market-outcomes

Sumner, A., Hoy, C. and Ortiz-Juarez, E. 2020. Estimates of the impact of COVID-19 on global poverty. WIDER Working Paper 2020/43. Helsinki: UNU-WIDER. https://doi.org/10.35188/UNU-WIDER/2020/800-9.

Web Desk. 2020. Parliament session: No data available on migrants' deaths during lockdown, says govt. *The Indian Express*, 14 September.

Part I

Law, Biomedical Emergencies, and Policy Response

1 Policing the Margins

Citizen–Police Interactions in India During COVID-19

Manjesh Rana

24 March 2020 marks the beginning of the first nationwide lockdown in India to contain the spread of COVID-19, which was arguably one of the most stringent lockdowns in the world. According to the COVID-19 stringency index, lockdown in India scored 100 per cent between 25 March 2020 and 19 April 2020, on a scale based on several indicators, including school closures, workplace closures, and travel bans.[1] A legal regime was put in place mainly under the Disaster Management Act, 2005, and the Epidemic Diseases Act, 1897, apart from orders under Section 144, the Code of Criminal Procedure, 1973.[2] The initial lockdown of three weeks was followed by several lockdowns with varied restrictions.

The global public health crisis caused unforeseen challenges to governance in the entire world. While the pandemic placed the public health agencies of every country at the forefront, after them, it was the law enforcement apparatus that took the biggest blow. The lockdown announced by the prime minister of India instantly restricted the movement of its 1.38 billion population. With only a four-hour window at hand, the announcement caught everyone unaware, including the police. The state governments, district administration, and the police had no time to put in necessary measures in place to ensure coordination and minimise the adversities for people while ensuring adequate compliance with the lockdown rules.

The lack of administrative planning and coordination, combined with the insufficient supply and support of essential services, caused chaos and confusion on the ground. The police in India had a difficult time reconciling with its new and emerging realities. Post-lockdown order, following a conventional 'law and order paradigm', the police agencies across the country aggressively enforced social distancing and other rules and regulations through patrolling vans, on-foot vigil, and vehicular checkpoints.[3] In addition, the pandemic also brought the police to the forefront of public health campaigns, with several other responsibilities at their disposal—from disseminating information about the nature of the virus to making people aware of the dos and don'ts amid chaos and uncertainty. The law enforcement institutions in all the states, thus, took an additional role—that of public health messengers.

DOI: 10.4324/9781003591641-3

Consequently, the pandemic brought police personnel into direct contact with common people in need of urgent help and assistance and modified, to a great extent, their primary role and the nature of duties performed by them during 'normal' times.

In addition, thousands of migrant workers, who were left stranded in desperate attempts to return to their home states, further added to the public order challenges of policing in India. Amid a sequence of unprecedented pandemic-induced lockdowns disrupting the social and economic structure, the kind of policing unleashed in the guise of controlling the situation was categorised among the worst impacts of the lockdown.[4]

Against this backdrop, the present chapter attempts to understand the facets of policing in India after the onset of COVID-19 by looking at varied aspects of the citizen–police interactions and the emergence of new challenges for the law enforcement apparatus, particularly when such interactions turned into violent confrontations. For the analysis, apart from several studies conducted during COVID-19, including the Commonwealth Human Rights Initiative's (CHRI's) review of reported accounts of police excesses,[5] the Criminal Justice & Police Accountability Project's (CPA Project's) study of sanctioned violence in the state of Madhya Pradesh,[6] the Gaon Connection-Lokniti rural report,[7] and several ground reports by media highlighting instances of police excess, it primarily uses the evidence collected through face-to-face interviews conducted by Lokniti—a Programme for Comparative Democracy at the Centre for the Study of Developing Societies (CSDS) and Common Cause among 2,409 civilians and 1,198 police personnel in 19 cities spread across 10 of the most affected states and union territories in India during the first wave of COVID-19 (hereinafter, 'the CSDS study').[8] The interviews were conducted face to face with the help of an Interview Schedule during October and November 2020.[9] A detailed method note is shared in the endnotes.[10]

Based on the empirical evidence of the CSDS study, the chapter makes three important observations—*first*, while police largely played a helpful and supportive role during pandemic-induced lockdowns, a significant proportion of police personnel proved to be inefficient in controlling situations like the COVID-19 pandemic owing to the lack of training and a basic humanitarian outlook; *second*, police in India often resorted to using humiliation or shame as a means to achieve their goal of making people abide by the ambiguous rules, with a significant proportion of them even using physical force; and *third*, socio-economically disadvantaged sections disproportionately bore the burden of police excesses, pushing them further to the margins.

1.1 Over-Policing During COVID-19-Induced Lockdowns

At the onset of COVID-19 in early 2020, policymakers around the globe found lockdown as the most immediate and proactive solution to curtail the spread of the deadly contagion. The Indian government too followed the dictum that 'prevention is better than cure'. This seemed like the primary measure, especially in the absence of any vaccination or medication. The burden of keeping the virus at bay, thus, had been disproportionally placed on common people, with an overt emphasis on preventing the spread of the contagion through certain behavioural and sanitation norms, such as the regular use of sanitiser and maintaining physical or social distance.[11] The suddenly declared lockdown, however, led to shock and panic among common people, forcing them to rush to their nearest shops and markets to hoard the essentials. The primary responsibility of settling this chaos came upon the local police, which, in the absence of clear guidelines, tightened the control over public spaces filled with panic-stricken citizens, resulting in several incidences of heavy-handed police actions against the 'violators'.[12]

Half of the police personnel interviewed in the CSDS study claimed to have frequently imposed fines and penalties on those who violated lockdown rules (Table 1.1). Amid general chaos and ambiguity about the rules and regulations, and in a situation where people were running from pillar to post to arrange for essentials, one can imagine the additional monetary burden imposed on them due to such fines that ranged from INR 200 to INR 3000. For instance, in November 2020, the Government of Delhi hiked the fine for not wearing a mask from INR 500 to INR 2000.[13] Similarly, in Pune, those found in violation of the mandatory use of face masks were imposed a fine of INR 500, while a repeat offender had to pay a fine up to INR 2000 (second time) and INR 3000 (third time).[14]

While the police can justify the collection of fines as the guidelines were being enforced under the Disaster Management Act of 2005, it went beyond their legal jurisdiction on several occasions. In the absence or lack of proper training to handle such unprecedented situations, and with arbitrary and discretionary powers in their hands due to ambiguous and inconsistent guidelines, the police often found themselves resorting to other means, such as leaving violators after giving them minor punishments, and at times, even using force on them to make them fall in the line. Throughout the lockdown, several cases were reported where the police tried to shame or humiliate those who were found in violation of the COVID-19 protocol, to set a precedent for others. A report released by the CHRI, which reviewed the reported accounts of police excesses, identified some of the most common extra-legal punishments given by the police during the lockdown.[15] The punishments included branding on the forehead and arms, posting selfies with derogatory captions, forcing people to carry placards, physical acts of humiliation, writing apology letters, and scaring violators with fake COVID-19 patients.[16]

For instance, in Meerut, Uttar Pradesh, the violators were made to hold up placards reading 'I am a friend of Coronavirus' or 'I am the enemy of society'.[17] Subsequently, their pictures were uploaded on Twitter (now X) and other social media platforms. In several other districts, people were also made to do sit-ups and squats by police as an instant punishment for breaking the lockdown rules. In one such incident, police personnel forced people to hop like frogs for being seen out on the road while the lockdown was in place.[18] Several media reports highlighted the brutality of police towards the violators, where they were seen beating civilians with batons.[19] Pictures and videos of people being brutally beaten up by police allegedly for breaking the lockdown rules emerged from all parts of the country.[20]

Looking at the empirical evidence, as highlighted in Table 1.1, one in every three police personnel who were part of the CSDS study agreed that they often gave 'minor punishments' to the violators before letting them go, while about the same proportion claimed to have humiliated the already horrified people 'a few times'. What's more, another one in three claimed to have used some kind of force on the violators 'very often' or 'a few times', while almost two in every five claimed to have even detained or arrested the violators on several occasions (Table 1.1).

In one such case, called 'India's George Floyd moment', a father-son duo, Jeyaraj and Bennicks, was arrested by the Tamil Nadu Police for allegedly violating the lockdown rules.[21] The two were remanded in the custody, and three days after the arrest, Bennicks died immediately after being admitted to the hospital, while his father died the next morning in similar circumstances. Following outrage by the public, the Central Bureau of Investigation (CBI) charged about 10 police personnel with murder, wrongful confinement, destruction of evidence, misconduct, and furnishing false evidence.[22]

The CHRI report of 2020 compiled as many as 150 incidences of police excesses starting from 24 March 2020 (the day India declared its first nationwide lockdown) until 31 May 2020, that is, within a span of a little over two months.[23] The instances highlighted police using physical force through beating, kicking, or *lathi*-charge as well as inflicting verbal abuse, insults, and degrading treatment on people, including essential service providers.[24] As per

Table 1.1 Half of the police personnel reported frequent penalisation of the violators during lockdown, and one in three personnel reported frequent use of force (%)

How Many Times Did You or Your Team Have to . . .	*Very Often*	*A Few Times*	*Rarely*	*Never*
Impose fine/penalty on the people who violated lockdown rules	50	24	10	14
Leave them after giving some minor punishment	34	32	13	17
Resort to the use of force	7	27	27	35
Detain/arrest them	12	25	25	35

Note: The remaining respondents did not answer. All figures are rounded off.

Source: SPIR 2020–2021, Vol. II, CSDS-Common Cause

Questions asked: During the last few months, how many times did you or your team had to do the following—very often, a few times, rarely, or never? a. Imposing fines/penalties on the people who violated lockdown rules; b. Leaving them after giving some minor punishment; c. Taking resort to the use of force; and d. Detaining/arresting them.

the CHRI report, more than 20 people, comprising mostly migrant workers and daily wage labourers, died in this period, following an interaction with the police. The brunt of police excesses was, thus, disproportionally borne by the socio-economically disadvantaged groups across the country.

In another case, a resident PG doctor, Hima Bindu, was assaulted by the police in Khammam district, Telangana, while she was out attending an emergency call of duty during lockdown at 8.30 pm.[25] Hima was initially stopped by a police constable and later taken to the local Additional Commissioner of Police (ACP), where she was verbally and physically assaulted despite explaining the emergency and producing her identity card. Narrating her ordeal, Hima shares the details of the assault:

> He (the ACP) asked me if I had any 'shame' and why was I out during the lockdown period despite being an 'educated girl'. I tried to reason out, but he slapped me and dragged me by my hair to the police station. There was no female police officer.[26]

The lockdown phase witnessed several similar stories, where even the ones providing essential services were subject to arbitrary police excesses. In response to a similar question in the CSDS study, while over one in every three people witnessed police using physical force, one in every ten witnessed police personnel using foul language when talking to the civilians (Table 1.2). Strengthening the argument, the evidence again indicates the

Table 1.2 Nearly one-third of citizens felt police were rude, and over one-third claimed they even used physical force (%)

	When the Lockdown Was in Place Did You Witness . . .	
	Use of Force on a Civilian by Police	*Police Speaking in a Rude Language*
Overall	*36*	*30*
Hindu Upper Castes	32	28
Hindu OBCs	37	32
Hindu Dalits	40	28
Hindu Adivasis*	41	36
Muslims	39	30
Christians^	37	30
Poor	39	31
Lower-class	35	31
Middle-class	38	27
Rich	32	29

*Note: The remaining respondents did not answer. All figures are rounded off. Relatively low sample size: *N = 66; ^N = 57.*

Source: SPIR 2020–2021, Vol. II, CSDS-Common Cause

Questions asked: When the lockdown was in place, did you witness any of the following: a. Police speaking in a rude language with people? and b. Use of force on a civilian by police?

socio-economically underprivileged sections to have been more at the receiving end of the brutality by the police. With about two in every five Hindu Dalits, Adivasis, and Muslims witnessing police resorting to forceful means against violators, such marginalised communities were about 10 percentage points more likely to be a victim of police excess than upper-caste Hindus. Similarly, those from poor households were significantly more likely to have witnessed police acting savagely.

Such arbitrary violence at the hands of police was not just wrong and illegal, but also counterproductive. Moreover, it indicates ill planning by the government at the centre, which instead of working with the states in finding the best practices for keeping people indoors, created a situation of panic, anxiety, and uncertainty. Hearing about an instant lockdown of as long as three weeks, it was expected that people would run to the nearest stores to hoard essentials, fearing and fighting both—the contagion and the police. With police being given total control of ensuring strict adherence to the lockdown rules, such incidences of arbitrary assaults by them further highlight the unpreparedness of the police in controlling situations like these.

Consequently, rather than looking at it as an act of care and protection, civilians were more likely to have felt threatened by the increased presence of police in their localities during the lockdown. This is evident by the fact that in the CSDS study almost three in every five of common people (combining 'a lot' and 'somewhat') claimed to be fearful of police imposing fines or penalties on them, while almost the same proportion feared that police would beat them up if they were found out of their homes to buy essentials or for work (Figure 1.1). What's more, a little over two in every five feared that police might forcefully take them to a hospital for Coronavirus testing or detain them in their custody.

Exploring the demographic differences, following a similar pattern, socio-economically disadvantaged sections were again found to be the most fearful. While 36 per cent of people belonging to rich households were found to be fearful of police beating them up, this proportion among poor households was as high as 58 per cent. Put simply, poor were over 1.5 times more fearful of the violence at the hands of police than the rich. Among those who were found to be fearful of police imposing fine, forcefully taking them to a hospital, and arresting them, the difference between rich and poor respondents was again significant, with the poor being at least 10 percentage points more fearful of police taking the aforementioned actions against them. What's more, as compared to the Hindu upper-caste communities, the Hindu OBCs, Dalits, and Adivasis were respectively 9, 13, and 16 percentage points more likely to be fearful of police beating them up.

The disproportionate burden of the COVID-19-induced restrictions on marginalised groups is also evident by the fact that a significant proportion of the general public in the CSDS study perceived the rules and regulations imposed during the lockdown to be unequal. On being asked if it was easy

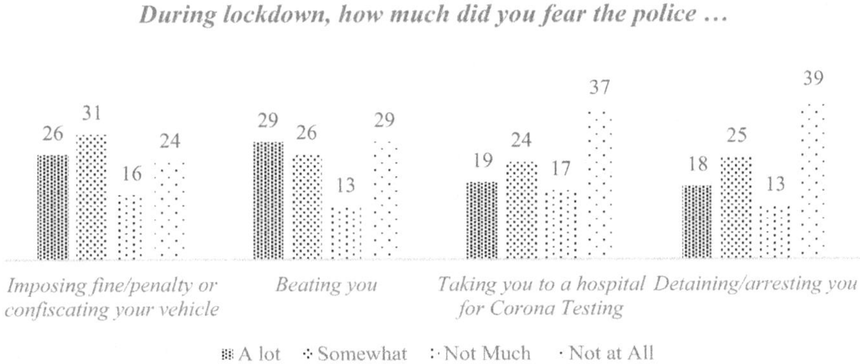

Figure 1.1 Over half of the civilians feared the imposition of a fine or use of physical force by the police during the lockdown (%)

Note: The rest of the respondents did not answer. All figures are rounded off.

Source: SPIR 2020–2021, Vol. II, CSDS-Common Cause

Questions asked: During the lockdown, whenever you went out of your home to buy essentials or for work, how much fear did you have of the following—a lot, somewhat, not much, or not at all? a. Fear of police imposing a fine/penalty or confiscating your vehicle? b. Fear of police beating you? c. Fear of police taking you to a hospital for testing? and d. Fear of police detaining/arresting you?

for some people to get away with the prohibitions imposed or whether the rules were the same for everyone, while over three-fifths of people felt they were the same for all, a significant proportion of nearly one-third felt that it was easier for some people to get away. Hinting at this economic divide, contrary to the rich cohorts, the poor were about 10 percentage points less likely to feel that everyone was treated equally. What's more, corroborating this viewpoint with another piece of evidence, over a quarter of police personnel who were part of the CSDS study echoed these sentiments and accepted that the rich sections of the society comfortably navigated through the strict lockdown rules.

The rich-poor divide during lockdown is validated through several other media reports and studies. According to the CPA Project' study conducted in the state of Madhya Pradesh, most of the lockdown-related complaints were filed against people on streets, mainly pedestrians and people on two-wheelers, showing an increase of about 50 per cent in the first lockdown and a whopping 90 per cent in the second lockdown.[27] This was followed by 'petty shopkeepers and street vendors', accounting for every fifth person against whom an FIR was filed in the state, with nearly half of them being the ones supplying essentials like groceries, vegetables, and meat and dairy products.[28]

Highlighting the social divide, the CPA Project' study revealed a disproportionate representation of Muslims among the total number of arrested persons (24.45%) and accused persons (21.5%) in the state during lockdown which has merely 6.57 per cent of Muslims in its population.[29] Notably, this was not just a lockdown phenomenon, as several reports have stressed the overrepresentation of backward classes and religious minorities across Indian prisons. Highlighting the social and economic vulnerability, the Death Penalty India Report of 2016 noted that about three in every four prisoners sentenced to death belonged to backward classes and religious minorities.[30]

1.2 The Plight of Migrant Workers

What was indeed a prelude to the 21-day lockdown, during the day-long '*Janata* curfew' just two days before the announcement, the government had already shut down the Indian Railways and the interstate bus service, leaving millions of migrants in the cities with dilemma and confusion.[31] Consequentially, post-lockdown, millions of migrants who were left stranded in the big cities were seen trudging towards their hometowns and villages.[32] As per a study conducted by Gaon Connection and Lokniti-CSDS among rural households in India after the first series of lockdowns, nearly a quarter of migrant workers (23%) returned home walking, while close to one-third (30%) returned by buses and trains.[33] What's more, for over two in every three migrant workers (67%), it took at least two days to return from the cities to their native villages, while over a fifth of migrant workers (21%) claimed to have spent at least five days in transit before reaching their homes.[34]

Against this backdrop, an important question arises—could a longer notice before the lockdown have prevented this unprecedented migrant crisis, or would that have defeated the sole purpose behind the lockdown?

While the Indian Council of Medical Research (ICMR) presumably had rational arguments to advise the Indian government to push the lockdown button, the evidence from the CSDS study reveals that about two in every three common people believed that a longer notice before the lockdown could have prevented such a large-scale migrant crisis. On the other hand, about one in three felt that a larger window would have been counterproductive. This perception was much stronger in the big Tier I cities like Delhi, Chennai, and Ahmedabad, which were at the centre of the pandemic at its onset and had witnessed a mass exodus of migrants post-lockdown. While three in every four of those living in Tier I cities believed the state should have given more time, in Tier II and III cities, three in every five felt so.

The official figure of internal migrants in India stood at over 45 billion in 2011—36 per cent of the population.[35] One can, therefore, imagine the plight of migrants who were left with no option but to walk hundreds of kilometres to reach their homes. On the other hand, one can also imagine the hardship faced by the police in taking control of the situation. The evidence from the CSDS study indicates that about three in every five police personnel were deployed to facilitate the homeward journey of stranded migrants during the first wave of COVID-19. On being asked about how difficult it was for them to control the migrants, overall, nearly two in every five of such police personnel found it 'extremely difficult' to manage the situation, while over two in every five found it 'somewhat difficult'.

Consequently, as the CSDS study further reveals, 7 in every 10 police personnel interviewed accepted using physical force to control the migrants walking towards their homes (Figure 1.2). Segregating this data further, one in every two cops resorted to using force against the helpless migrant workers 'a few times' or 'very often'. On the other hand, only about a quarter of police personnel denied using force against migrant groups during the lockdown.

Further revealing the atrocities by police on the helpless migrants, a significant proportion of migrant workers (12%) interviewed in the Gaon Connection-CSDS rural study claimed to have been beaten by the cops while returning to their homes.[36]

What's more, in a rapid survey,[37] which was a part of the CSDS study, conducted separately among aid workers and migrant workers, nearly a fifth of migrant workers claimed to have either been assaulted by the police or frequently come across someone who had been a victim of police excesses during the lockdown. In response to another question, a significant proportion (9%) of migrant workers claimed to have faced physical assault by the police while attempting to return to their homes. Sharing one such narrative of police high-handedness from the rapid survey:

> Mahesh (name changed) is a 24-year-old migrant worker from Ganjam Odisha who was working in Surat, Gujarat, as an industry worker, earning a salary of INR 16,000 before the lockdown. He and his brother left for their village from Surat on 26 May 2020 by train through an agent. He and his brother had to take a bus to the station. The bus stop was crowded and they were afraid of missing the train. When they

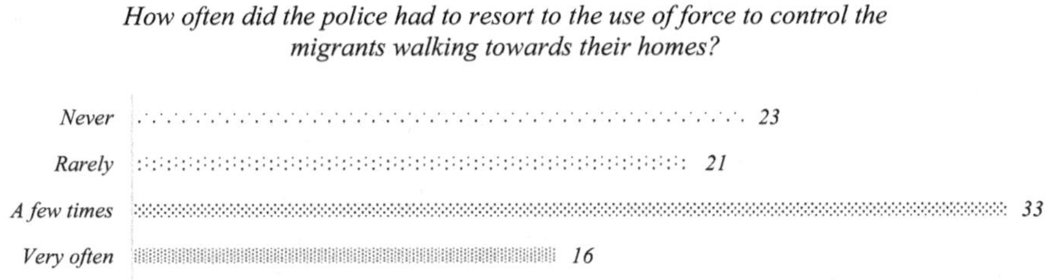

Figure 1.2 Half of the police personnel reported the use of force against migrants travelling back home during the lockdown (%)

Note: The rest of the respondents did not answer. All figures are rounded off.

Source: SPIR 2020–2021, Vol. II, CSDS-Common Cause

Question asked: How often did the police have to resort to the use of force to control the migrants walking towards their homes—very often, a few times, rarely, or never?

attempted to board the bus, the police started beating them. The police was hitting everyone indiscriminately. In the confusion, when Mahesh turned to look for his brother he found him lying on the ground. He was rushed to the hospital where they pronounced him dead on arrival. Despite Mahesh and his family's insistence for a post-mortem, the police refused. Mahesh was forced to cremate his brother in Surat. Since he had no money to return to his village, some acquaintances booked a ticket for him and he managed to return home.[38]

1.3 Police: Understaffed, Overburdened, and Undertrained

The task of managing such an unprecedented exodus of migrants amid the chaos and uncertainty due to the suddenly declared lockdown was never expected to be an easy one for the police that already suffered from several existing issues, including having acutely inadequate strength and lack of training or expertise of handling such a crisis, among many others.

The shortage of police personnel is a potential hurdle in the day-to-day discharge of duties by the police. According to the data shared by the Bureau of Police Research and Development (BPR&D),[39] as of 1 January 2020, the police in India worked at 79.7 per cent of its sanctioned strength, that is, at four-fifths of its required strength.[40] Put differently, there are only 155 cops for every 100,000 Indian citizens, as against 195 sanctioned posts (a vacancy of 20%). This makes India's police force one of the most understaffed and weakest in the world, lagging far behind most of the countries in the world and the United Nations' recommended ratio of 222.[41]

Notably, policing being a state subject, there is a significant variation across different Indian states. The 'actual police' to 'sanctioned police' ratio (in percentages) at the onset of the pandemic for the 10 states where the CSDS study was conducted is highlighted in Figure 1.3. While states like Tamil Nadu, Delhi, and Maharashtra had vacancies between 10 and 12 per cent, Bihar and West Bengal featured at the bottom, with over one-third vacancies for police personnel. This added further to the hardship caused while managing the pandemic-induced lockdowns.

Corroborating this, on being asked about the challenges faced by them during the COVID-19 pandemic, over half of the police personnel interviewed in the CSDS study accepted facing difficulties due to a shortage of staff while fighting the outbreak (Table 1.3). Besides this, a quarter of police personnel identified the confusion among themselves regarding who needed to arrange for shelter for stranded migrants to be another major challenge for them during the time. What's more, while nearly the same proportion claimed a lack of coordination with police from other districts or regions to be very challenging, one-fifth of police personnel also reported the shortage of funds to be a major hurdle.

The issue of perpetual vacancies worsens several other connected problems of overworked and overburdened police, which is the root cause of

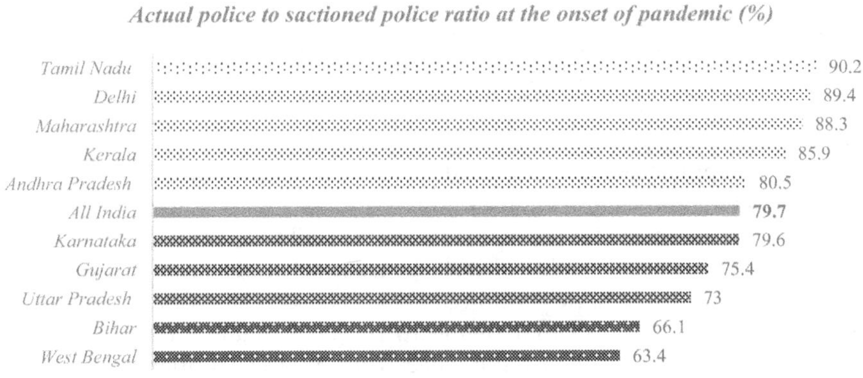

Figure 1.3 Overall, the Indian police work at four-fifths of their sanctioned strength; and in a few states, there are as high as one-third vacancies

Note: The chart highlights the actual-to-sanctioned ratio of total police, including civil police, armed reserve police, special armed police, and Indian reserve battalion as of 1 January 2020 in the 10 states where the CSDS study was conducted.

Source: BPR&D, Ministry of Home Affairs, 2020

Table 1.3 Over half of the police personnel admitted facing difficulties due to a shortage of staff (%)

Challenges Faced by Police While Fighting COVID-19	
Shortage of staff	52
Confusion regarding who needed to arrange for shelter for stranded migrants	23
Lack of coordination with police from other districts/regions	22
Lack of financial resources	19

Note: All figures are rounded off.

Source: SPIR 2020–2021, Vol. II

Questions asked: In your experience, did the police in this locality face any of the following while fighting the Coronavirus outbreak: a. Lack of financial resources; b. Shortage of staff; c. Lack of coordination with police from other districts/regions; and d. Confusion regarding who needed to arrange for shelter for stranded migrants?

both physical and mental stress among police personnel.[42] Consequently, the working hours for the police increased significantly during the first wave. Owing to several additional tasks assigned to the police force and the existing problem of shortage of staff, close to four in every five police personnel had to be on duty for at least 11 hours a day. Notably, even during the 'normal times', that is, before the lockdown was announced, over three-fifths of police personnel reported working such long hours daily. What's more, a quarter of police personnel reported working at least 15 hours a day during the lockdown. The police in metropolitan cities like Delhi, Kolkata, and Chennai were found far more exhausted in this regard, with 9 in every 10 of them reportedly working for at least 11 hours a day.

One can also imagine the physical and mental toll on the health of personnel bound to the call of their duty despite the fear of the virus. The evidence from the CSDS study indicates that for over two-fifths of police personnel, being on regular duty during the COVID-19 outbreak severely impacted their mental health. Exhaustion and fear were such that if they had a choice, two in every five police personnel would have taken a leave and stayed at home for their safety and that of their family.

Lastly, in addition to the existing responsibilities, the pandemic added several tasks to the portfolio of police personnel that would have required specialised and systematic training. Over half of the police personnel in the CSDS study reported that owing to the challenging circumstances and unprecedented tasks at their hand, special training was imparted to them to deal with the common public. However, on the other hand, over two-fifths denied receiving any such training. Put simply, at least two police personnel in every five were out in the field, trying to manage the unprecedented situation created due to COVID-19, without any specialised knowledge and training.

Given how quickly the virus spread, one might believe that it was rather extremely difficult to provide specific and specialised training to such a large force to deal with an unprecedented pandemic-like situation, with no time in hand. In such a scenario, it would perhaps make more sense to see how well our police force is trained in other aspects of policing, which are part of a routine exercise. Several training modules are designed for police personnel to impart multiple standard and practical skills, making them aware of international standards for human rights, as well as sensitizing them towards different vulnerable groups. A 2019 pan-India study by CSDS and Common Cause, conducted among police personnel, highlighted the status of three kinds of training—human rights, caste sensitisation, and crowd control—all of which proved highly important in handling the COVID-19-induced lockdowns.[43]

Firstly, as revealed in the 2019 study, two in every five cops (41%) received the essential training about human rights only at the time of joining, while a significant proportion of police personnel (12%) never received such training.[44] On the other hand, only a quarter police force (25%) received their training in human rights during the last two to three years.[45]

Secondly, showing a similar trend, nearly half (45%) of the police force received training about caste sensitisation only once in their time of service, that is, only at the time they joined the police force, while 11 per cent of them never received it.

Lastly, the 2019 study also revealed that one in every two police personnel (51%) received training in crowd control only at the time of their joining, while a small portion of 4 per cent never received it. With only 3 in every 10 police personnel (30%) provided with essential training in crowd control in the last two to three years, one can imagine the level of unpreparedness on the part of the police, especially in dealing with the chaos and panic among public created due to the suddenly declared lockdown.[46]

What's more, looking at state-wise variations, Bihar fared worst in training their police force in human rights, with about two in every five cops (38%) who have never received such training, followed by Assam (31%) and Gujarat (30%). Further, looking at the training about caste sensitisation, one in every four cops in Assam (27%), Kerala (27%), Bihar (24%), and Gujarat (24%) claimed to have never received such training. Lastly, even though states fared relatively better in training their force in crowd control, in Assam, nearly one in every five police personnel (18%) never received such training, and in Bihar, while 7 in every 10 (69%) received it only at the time of joining, 11 per cent of them are still to be trained.[47] Notably, Bihar had the second biggest share of migrant workers who returned to the state during lockdown—12 per cent—while Gujarat feature among the top four states that house over half of the country's interstate migrants.[48]

1.4 Conclusion

With an unprecedented pandemic at the backdrop, police were seen as a crucial interface between the state and its citizens across the world.[49] While it is true that the police personnel had to reinvent themselves to a large extent and assume a new and far more challenging role to tackle panic-stuck citizens, the absence of specialised training to handle pandemic-like situations, lack of readiness among the police force owing to a suddenly declared lockdown, prejudices against socio-economically vulnerable groups, and the existing infrastructural challenges put the Indian police force across the states in a position of great disadvantage.

The shreds of evidence from the CSDS study, combined with other ground reports, exposed serious deficiencies in policing in India. The empirical findings indicate that in the absence of proper and well-established guidelines and Standard Operating Procedures (SOPs) delineating measures for carrying out new tasks during the COVID-19-induced lockdown, the police did not shy away from using their powers arbitrarily against the citizens, with the socio-economically disadvantaged sections, migrant workers, and marginalised communities disproportionately bearing the burden of 'over-policing'.

Shaming and humiliating people against the backdrop of a public health emergency and the use of repressive force against them for breaking the lockdown rules indicate an acute lack of compassion among police personnel and an instinctual reflex towards the use of violence. A significant proportion of the police force also seemed to be unfamiliar with or chose to ignore the globally accepted norms guiding the use of force by police, having internalised the 'macho' or expedient way of dealing with things.[50]

While some of the problems with policing in India, which persist due to pre-existing ailments in the system—like the police being understaffed, overburdened, underfunded, and undertrained—have been highlighted by the reformers time and again, COVID-19 further widened these gaps, calling the attention of the state towards putting safeguards in place, institutionalising accountability and minimising the instances of police excesses. The overt dependence on the use of excessive force points out the failure of police to quickly adapt and articulate a systematic plan to respond to the sudden lockdown.[51]

The gruelling ordeal of Indian police, which seems to be a perennial issue across the country, stresses the urgent need for filling the vacant posts and increasing the sanctioned strength of the police. COVID-19 also enforced the need to regularly impart the necessary training to the police personnel, making them more efficient while navigating through challenging circumstances, as well as making them sensitive towards vulnerable groups. With the threat of another wave of the contagion always around the corner, it makes absolute sense to design specialised training modules and SOPs to help police personnel deal with a similar situation in the future more systematically and strategically.

List of Abbreviations

ACP	Additional Commissioner of Police
BHK	Bedroom, Hall, and Kitchen
BPR&D	Bureau of Police Research and Development
CBI	Central Bureau of Investigation
CHRI	Commonwealth Human Rights Initiative
CPA Project	Criminal Justice and Police Accountability Project
COVID-19	Coronavirus Disease of 2019
CrPC	Criminal Procedure Code
CSDS	Centre for the Study of Developing Societies
FIR	First Information Report
ICMR	Indian Council of Medical Research
INR	Indian Rupee
NCT	National Capital Territory
OBCs	Other Backward Classes
SOPs	Standard Operating Procedures
SPIR	Status of Policing in India Report
SPSS	Statistical Package for the Social Sciences
UT	Union Territory
Vol.	Volume

Notes

1 *Covid-19 Government Response Tracker*, Blavatnik School of Government, University of Oxford, 2020. Accessed 26 June 2024. www.bsg.ox.ac.uk/research/research-projects/covid-19-government-response-tracker.

2 Section 144 of the Criminal Procedure Code (CrPC) of 1973 authorises the Executive Magistrate of any state or territory to issue an order to prohibit the assembly of four or more people in an area.

3 Akshay Mangla, and Vineet Kapoor, How policing works in India in covid-19 times, *Business Line*, 2 June 2020. Accessed 25 May 2022. www.thehindubusinessline.com/opinion/columns/how-policing-works-in-india-in-covid-19-times/article31729922.ece.

4 *Policing During India's Covid-19 Lockdown: A Review of Reported Accounts of Police Excesses*, New Delhi: Commonwealth Human Rights Initiatives (CHRI), 2020. Accessed 13 August 2022. www.humanrightsinitiative.org/download/1616584225Policing%20during%20lockdown.pdf.

5 *Policing During India's Covid-19 Lockdown: A Review of Reported Accounts of Police Excesses*, New Delhi: Commonwealth Human Rights Initiatives (CHRI), 2020. Accessed 13 August 2022. www.humanrightsinitiative.org/download/1616584225Policing%20during%20lockdown.pdf.

6 *Countermapping Pandemic Policing: A Study of Sanctioned Violence in Madhya Pradesh*, Bhopal: Criminal Justice & Police Accountability Project (CPA Project). Accessed 25 June 2024. https://cpaproject.in/wp-content/uploads/2023/08/Countermapping-Pandemic-Policing-CPAProject.pdf.

7 *The Rural Report: Impact of Covid-19 on Rural India*, Lucknow: Gaon Connection, 2020. Accessed 29 January 2023. www.gaonconnection.com/h-library/final-rural-report-2020-updated.pdf.

8 *Status of Policing in India Report (SPIR) 2020–2021: Vol. II Policing in the Covid-19 Pandemic*, New Delhi: Lokniti-Centre for the Study of Developing Societies (CSDS) and Common Cause, 2021. Accessed 29 January 2022. https://lokniti.org/media/upload_files/SPIR%202020-2021_Vol.%20II_Full%20Report_Aug%206.pdf. The author was the Project Coordinator and Lead Researcher for the study.

9 The study was conducted during the months of October and November in 2020, and therefore it is confined to the first wave of COVID-19 and the first phase of the consequential lockdown(s) that were imposed in 2020.

10 Method note: The present chapter uses evidence from the study 'Status of Policing in India Report 2020–21: Policing in Covid-19 Pandemic' which is based on a sample survey of 3607 individuals (1198 police personnel and 2409 civilians), across 19 cities of 10 states/union territories of India. The survey, which comprises face-to-face interviews with the respondents at the place of work or residence of the respondent using a standardized questionnaire in the language spoken and understood by them, was conducted by Lokniti- CSDS and Common Cause in October and November 2020. The fieldwork was conducted strictly following the COVID-19 protocol. The following Indian states (and cities) were shortlisted—Andhra Pradesh (Visakhapatnam and East Godavari), Bihar (Patna and Muzaffarpur), Gujarat (Ahmedabad and Surat), Karnataka (Bengaluru and Bellary), Kerala (Thiruvananthapuram and Mallapuram), Maharashtra (Pune and Nashik), Tamil Nadu (Chennai and Thiruvallur), The NCT of Delhi, Uttar Pradesh (Lucknow and Kanpur Nagar), and West Bengal (Kolkata and North 24 Parganas). Eight of these feature among the 10 most-affected states during the pandemic, that is, having the highest number of COVID-19 cases as of 15 August 2020, while the other two are Gujarat (for being one of the worst-hit states due to the migrant crisis) and Kerala (for being one of the earliest regions to have been hit by COVID-19). One Tier I city and one Tier II or III city with the maximum number of COVID-19 cases as of 15 August 2020 have been selected from each of the states for the study. In states which do not have a Tier I city, the two most affected Tier II or III cities were selected. A total of 360 interviews (120 interviews of the police personnel and 240 interviews of the civilians) were

targeted from each of the 10 states/Union Territories in the sample. In every sampled city, two to three locations were shortlisted in each of the four different regions within the city—North, East, South, and West. Priority was given to those locations that were relatively more affected by the pandemic. Interviews were also conducted in the market/trading areas and some other public spaces where citizen–police interaction was more likely to occur frequently. For civilians, within a particular locality, the interviews were taken from all types of localities—poor, lower class, middle class, and rich. The sample was divided in the following proportion across the four types of localities— poor (slums/jhuggis/basti/shanties): 20 per cent; lower class (houses with just one to two rooms or one BHK houses/flats/apartments): 40 per cent; middle class (three BHK houses/flats/apartments): 30 per cent; and rich (four BHK houses/flats/apartments, independent bungalows, and posh colonies): 10 per cent. Ensuring that the sample is spread across all the houses/streets/colonies in a given location, depending on the size of the locality, a person was interviewed in every third or fifth house. To make the sample representative, the targeted male-female ratio was equal, that is, 50:50, while the targeted age-wise proportion of the respondents was as follows: 18–25 years: 25 per cent; 26–35 years: 25 per cent; 36–45 years: 20 per cent; 46–55 years: 14 per cent; and 56 years and above; 16 per cent. Only persons of minimum of 18 years of age were interviewed. For police personnel, interviews were conducted at police stations, police chowkis, police booths, and various other places where the police personnel were deployed. The locations chosen for the police personnel's interviews were the same as those for the civilians. As far as it was possible, the male-female ratio among police respondents was maintained at 80:20, that is, 80 per cent of the total interviews were conducted with the male police personnel, while 20 percent interviews were conducted with the female police personnel. Further, as far as feasible, the targeted ratio of 'Constabulary-Rank Officers' to 'High-Rank Officers' was maintained at 80:20, that is, 80 per cent of the police personnel of constabulary ranks and 20 per cent from the higher ranks were targeted for the interviews. The analyses presented in the chapter have been done using Statistical Package for the Social Sciences (SPSS).

11 T. K. Rajalakshmi, Deficient system, *The Frontline*, 22 March 2020. Accessed 27 June 2024. https://frontline.thehindu.com/cover-story/article31130768.ece.

12 Jasmitha Arvind, and Vinita Govindarajan, Coronavirus: India's lockdown has led to chaos because the Government misunderstood how cities work, *Scroll.in*, 10 April 2020. Accessed 25 November 2022. https://scroll.in/article/958140/coronavirus-indias-lockdown-has-led-to-chaos-because-the-government-misunderstood-how-cities-work.

13 How states are penalising public for violating Covid-19 rules, *The Indian Express*, 21 November 2020. Accessed 25 May 2022. https://indianexpress.com/article/india/states-fines-violating-coronavirus-covid-19-mask-social-distancing-rules-7060100/.

14 How states are penalising public for violating Covid-19 rules, *The Indian Express*, 21 November 2020. Accessed 25 May 2022. https://indianexpress.com/article/india/states-fines-violating-coronavirus-covid-19-mask-social-distancing-rules-7060100/.

15 *Policing During India's Covid-19 Lockdown*, CHRI.

16 *Policing During India's Covid-19 Lockdown*, CHRI.

17 Saurabh Sharma, Friend of coronavirus: Police in North India shame those defying lockdown, *Reuters*, 24 March 2020. Accessed 25 May 2022. www.reuters.com/article/us-health-coronavirus-india-police-idUSKBN21B23Z.

18 Anisha Sircar, India's coronavirus lockdown is bringing out the worst in its police force, *Quartz*, 28 March 2022. Accessed 19 September 2022. https://qz.com/india/1826387/indias-coronavirus-lockdown-brings-police-brutality-to-the-fore.

19 Indian police use force against coronavirus lockdown offenders, *Aljajeera*, 30 March 2020. Accessed 12 May 2022. www.aljazeera.com/program/newsfeed/2020/3/30/indian-police-use-force-against-coronavirus-lockdown-offenders.
20 Rohan Venkataramakrishnan, The Indian police must understand that coronavirus cannot be beaten with a lathi, *Scroll.in*, 26 March 2020. Accessed 29 June 2022. https://scroll.in/article/957269/the-indian-police-need-to-understand-that-coronavirus-cannot-be-beaten-with-a-lathi.
21 Swati Gupta, and Julia Hollingsworth, They were arrested for breaking lockdown rules. Then they died in police custody, *CNN*, 2 July 2020. Accessed 12 August 2022. https://edition.cnn.com/2020/07/01/asia/tamil-nadu-deaths-custody-intl-hnk/index.html.
22 Mohit Rao, Indian police use violence as a shortcut to justice. It's the poorest who bear the scars, *CNN*, 3 December 2020. Accessed 12 August 2022. https://edition.cnn.com/2020/12/02/india/police-brutality-india-dst-intl-hnk/index.html.
23 *Policing During India's Covid-19 Lockdown*, CHRI.
24 *Policing During India's Covid-19 Lockdown*, CHRI.
25 Rishika Sadam, What good are claps? Hero doctors on virus duty slapped by cops, kicked out of homes, called 'dirty', *News18*, 25 March 2020. Accessed 29 October 2022. www.news18.com/news/india/whats-the-use-of-claps-hero-doctors-slapped-by-cops-kicked-out-of-homes-called-dirty-over-virus-duty-2549987.html.
26 Rishika Sadam, What good are claps? Hero doctors on virus duty slapped by cops, kicked out of homes, called 'dirty', *News18*, 25 March 2020. Accessed 29 October 2022. www.news18.com/news/india/whats-the-use-of-claps-hero-doctors-slapped-by-cops-kicked-out-of-homes-called-dirty-over-virus-duty-2549987.html.
27 *Countermapping Pandemic Policing*, CPA Project.
28 *Countermapping Pandemic Policing*, CPA Project.
29 *Countermapping Pandemic Policing*, CPA Project.
30 *Death Penalty India Report*, New Delhi: National Law University Delhi, 2016. Accessed 2 June 2022. www.project39a.com/dpir.
31 After trains, interstate bus services suspended till 31st March, *The Economic Times*, 22 March 2020. Accessed 25 May 2022. https://economictimes.indiatimes.com/news/politics-and-nation/after-trains-interstate-bus-services-suspended-till-31st-march/articleshow/74758323.cms.
32 Shoaib Daniyal, Not China, not Italy: India's coronavirus lockdown is the harshest in the world, *Scroll.in*, 10 April 202. Accessed 25 May 2022. https://scroll.in/article/957564/not-china-not-italy-indias-coronavirus-lockdown-is-the-harshest-in-the-world.
33 *The Rural Report*, Gaon Connection.
34 *The Rural Report*, Gaon Connection.
35 *Census of India*, Government of India, 2011. Accessed 25 May 2022. https://censusindia.gov.in/nada/index.php/catalog/42597.
36 *The Rural Report*, Gaon Connection.
37 Rapid Survey was conducted separately by the Common Cause as part of the 'SPIR 2020–2021'. The survey was conducted in parts of the Delhi-NCR region, Gujarat, and Rajasthan. For the survey, over 200 respondents (100 migrant workers and 114 aid workers) were interviewed in September 2020.
38 *SPIR 2020–2021*, CSDS and Common Cause.
39 *Data on Police Organisations*, New Delhi: Bureau of Police Research and Development (BPR&D), Ministry of Home Affairs, 2020. Accessed 25 June 2024. https://bprd.nic.in/uploads/dopo/dopo2020.pdf; *237th Report on Police-Training, Modernisation and Reforms*, New Delhi: Department-Related Parliamentary Standing Committee on Home Affairs, Rajya Sabha, 2022. Accessed 25 May 2022. https://rajyasabha.nic.in/rsnew/Committee_site/Committee_File/ReportFile/15/161/237_2022_2_17.pdf.

40 The figures presented here are of total police strength, which includes civil police, armed reserve police, special armed police, and Indian reserve battalion.
41 Sriharsha Devulapalli, and Vishnu Padmanabhan, India's police force among the world's weakest, *Mint*, 19 June 2019. Accessed 29 October 2022. www.livemint.com/news/india/india-s-police-force-among-the-world-s-weakest-1560925355383.html.
42 Bryan Vila, Impact of long work hours on police officers and the communities they serve, *American Journal of Industrial Medicine* 49 (11) (2006): 972–80.
43 *Status of Policing in India Report (SPIR) 2019: Police Adequacy and Working Conditions*, New Delhi: CSDS and Common Cause, 2019: 117–19. Accessed 14 May 2022. www.lokniti.org/archivetiles/spir_2019.
44 *Status of Policing in India Report (SPIR) 2019: Police Adequacy and Working Conditions*, New Delhi: CSDS and Common Cause, 2019: 117–19. Accessed 14 May 2022. www.lokniti.org/archivetiles/spir_2019.
45 The percentage includes 8 per cent of police personnel who joined the police force during the last three years.
46 The percentage includes 8 per cent of police personnel who joined the police force during the last three years.
47 *SPIR 2019*, CSDS and Common Cause.
48 Radheshyam Jadhav, Five states account for 67% migrant workers who returned home during the lockdown, *Business Line*, 11 February 2021. Accessed 3 August 2022. www.thehindubusinessline.com/data-stories/data-focus/five-states-account-for-67-migrant-workers-who-returned-home-during-the-lockdown/article33813158.ece; What the 2011 census data on migration tells us, *Hindustan Times*, 26 July 2019. Accessed 3 August 2022. www.hindustantimes.com/delhi-news/migration-from-up-bihar-disproportionately-high/story-K3WAio8TrrvBhd22VbAPLN.html.
49 Manjesh Rana, Threat, fear were most common police tools during Covid lockdown, study finds, *The Print*, 25 August 2021. Accessed 17 October 2022. https://theprint.in/opinion/threat-fear-were-most-common-police-tools-during-covid-lockdown-study-finds/721616/.
50 N. C. Asthana, Policing during India's Covid-19 lockdown, CHRI; Why police brutality and torture are endemic in India, *The Wire*, 13 December 2021. Accessed 12 May 2022. https://thewire.in/government/why-police-brutality-and-torture-are-endemic-in-india.
51 *Policing During India's Covid-19 Lockdown*, CHRI.

2 India's Fumbled COVID-19 Vaccine Policy

Nishant Sirohi

2.1 Introduction: People's Health in India

Healthcare in India has always trailed long behind the needs of the country; there is always a silent health crisis. Issues related to the availability, affordability and non-discriminatory access to healthcare facilities and essential medicines[1] continue to plague India's public healthcare system. Successive governments have failed to increase public health expenditure, which remains around 1 per cent of the GDP—one of the lowest in the world.[2] While India has improved its infant and maternal mortality rate[3] and life expectancy,[4] its health indicators continue to place it in the bottom quartile of the Human Development Index, ranking 134 out of 193 in 2023–2024.[5]

The Constitution of India does not accord a fundamental right to health, nor is there any legislation that envisages a right to health. Consequently, claims related to health, such as access to healthcare, essential medicines, and treatment, remain poorly understood and weakly protected. In the absence of a justiciable claim, decades of health rights litigation in India have nudged the courts to stand up for human dignity and construct a right-to-health framework within the fundamental right to life under Article 21 of the Constitution. As per the constitutional scheme, state governments are responsible for "public health and sanitation; hospitals and dispensaries".[6] However, the framing and financing of health policy has remained at the whim of the Union Government, which holds fiscal powers and heads the Central Council of Health and Family Welfare, the primary advisory and policymaking body on healthcare in India.[7] The fiscal centralisation of public health continues to strain India's cooperative federalism and often impinges upon the constitutional rights of state governments, even in times of crisis. For instance, not only are the policy decisions taken by the state governments are subject to the political orientation of the Union Government but the state governments have to also comply with the Union Government's unilateral directives.

This was particularly evident in India's response to the COVID-19 pandemic. In the absence of clear and comprehensive health legislation and framework which affirms rights and duties related to health and prepares to respond to severe epidemics, the Union Government was able to side-line

DOI: 10.4324/9781003591641-4

the state governments and use the obsolete Disaster Management Act, 2005[8] to frame its ad hoc and authoritarian policy responses to the COVID-19 pandemic. As the pandemic raged, the Union Government's policy responses to the pandemic became entirely disjointed,[9] resulting in what many have called a "policy-driven catastrophe".[10] More than the pandemic itself, the flawed actions of the Union Government and its subsequent attempts to minimise its obligation to deal with the pandemic caused adverse outcomes and irreversible damage. This policy incoherence was widely visible in India's COVID-19 vaccine strategy, which was tweaked by the Union Government several times[11]—until the Supreme Court of India intervened to align it with the constitutional scheme.

This chapter maps out the challenges in India's COVID-19 vaccine policy, which failed to ensure adequate vaccine availability and access for the most marginalised communities. Even though socio-economic rights are not justiciable under the Indian Constitution, the courts have evolved a jurisprudence that presents a framework to enforce the right to health in India. However, in framing the COVID-19 vaccine policy, the Government failed to consider the judicial directives related to access to healthcare, treatment and essential medicines. Instead of operationalising the jurisprudential framework, the Government relied on the inappropriate DMA, 2005, to frame its policy responses to the pandemic. As a result, the response to the pandemic was unnecessarily authoritarian, ad hoc and inconsistent. It exacerbated the devastating second wave, which wrecked lives across classes and castes but most disproportionately impacted the marginalised communities.[12]

Based on this discussion, the paper argues that addressing health issues superficially through public policy provisions and executive decisions is insufficient to improve the persistent systemic failures in the Indian healthcare system. The legal and constitutional basis for a right to health, repeatedly affirmed by the courts, must be solidified through legislative action. The COVID-19 pandemic did not precipitate a health crisis; it simply exposed the crisis that was always there.

2.2 Governance in the Crisis

> "[The] State has failed in fulfilling its obligations of protecting a basic Fundamental Right, i.e. Right to Life acknowledged in Article 21 of the Constitution of India".[13]
>
> —Delhi High Court

This observation from the Delhi High Court came on 30 April 2021 in a petition filed by a COVID-19 patient seeking the court's assistance in securing an ICU bed. The patient died before his case was heard.[14] This statement precisely summed up the crisis precipitated by the COVID-19 pandemic in India. During the virulent second wave, catastrophe struck as the Indian

State melted away,[15] and people were abandoned to their own devices and fate. Many died inside and outside hospitals across India, waiting for oxygen, medicines and hospital beds.[16] Social media was inundated with images and reports of overflowing crematoriums[17] and unclaimed bodies floating in the Ganges or buried in the dirt on its banks.[18] In this calamity, there was no human dignity in life, in passing away, or even after death.

The COVID-19 pandemic caught India, like the rest of the world,[19] poorly prepared. The pandemic sent shockwaves that shattered India's fragile healthcare infrastructure, which, even before the pandemic, was plagued by structural inequalities[20] and decades of underfunding. The pandemic caught India off-guard without a robust legal and policy framework to prepare for and respond to a public health emergency of this magnitude.[21] Despite its own failures, the Union Government responded to the pandemic with an iron fist. Snowden's scholarly work has demonstrated[22] how "a pandemic can lead to an illegal regime and excessive exercise of power over the citizens".[23] In India, the Union Government's policy responses to the pandemic were undemocratic. The Union Government and the state governments stretched available legal provisions from the DMA, 2005, and the Epidemic Disease Act, 1897[24] (EDA 1897), to legally substantiate their executive orders,[25] which severely restricted personal liberties.[26]

The DMA, 2005, was enacted primarily for natural disasters like earthquakes, floods and cyclones, granting sweeping powers to the central executive. Similarly, the archaic EDA, 1897, enacted by the British colonial regime in India during the bubonic plague, grants similar sweeping powers to state governments. Both these statutes effectively give the executive unrestricted rule-making powers with minimal parliamentary scrutiny.[27] Using these powers, the Union Government issued a slew of incoherent measures, including implementing the most stringent nationwide lockdown[28] with four hours' notice,[29] enforcing invasive surveillance measures without any data regulation policy in place[30] and suppressing democratic rights by cracking down on dissenters.[31]

A crisis tests a state's actual capacity to govern, the efficacy of its public policies and the quality of its governance. The Union Government's complacency was visible throughout the pandemic and exposed its acute failure to comprehend the gravity of the public health emergency.[32] For example, just before the second wave, the Union Government sent mixed messages about the endgame of the pandemic being in sight in India, and the public authorities failed to control mass political and religious gatherings,[33] which contributed to India's COVID-19 second wave.

The State is responsible for protecting the nation's integrity and the fundamental rights of all its citizens.[34] As defined in Article 12, the State includes the Government and the Parliament of India, the legislatures and Government of each state and local and "other authorities" within the jurisdiction of the Government of India. The Constitution grants the State an "enormous reservoir of prerogative and discretionary power"[35] to expand and exercise its executive muscle to handle extraordinary situations. Additionally, the Constitution, through the Directive Principles of State Policy (DPSPs), also provides a blueprint for governance with a sense of compassion and fraternity.[36] Article 38 commands the State to "eliminate inequalities in status, facilities and opportunities" and prohibits the "concentration of wealth and means of production to the common detriment".

The rationality and history of the Indian Constitution reflect that the fundamental rights and liberties mirror the basic values of the Indian people[37] and are derived from the normative promises of dignity and equality under the Constitution. These rights are also basic human rights[38] and cannot be taken away even by a constitutional amendment.[39] However, the fundamental guarantees—except Articles 20 and 21, which cannot be suspended under any circumstances[40]—can be subject to "reasonable restrictions" in the interest of society and the nation[41] and can only be suspended through a formal proclamation of emergency.[42] Any such restrictive measures taken by the State during a state of emergency should fulfil the objective of proportionality[43] and must be non-discriminatory.[44]

The COVID-19 pandemic inflicted an unprecedented humanitarian crisis, forcing the Union Government to take extraordinary measures to protect public health. However, even in a public health emergency, the State cannot bargain away fundamental rights. The policy measures and restrictive regulations enforced by the Union Government should have respected human rights and satisfy the constitutional prerequisite of proportionality.[45] It is pertinent to note that the Union Government did not proclaim an emergency. Instead, it single-handedly managed the entire pandemic, with some exceptions, through executive orders with no checks and balances from the legislative and judiciary. This measure taken by the Union Government brought the country back to the pre-44th Constitution Amendment era, where the decision-making powers rested solely with the executive and the legislative and judiciary remained static.[46]

The pandemic exposed India's healthcare vulnerabilities and the need for a cohesive policy framework. The inconsistent response to the pandemic worsened the crisis. A comprehensive COVID-19 vaccine policy was critical to mitigate health and economic fallout. However, challenges in its formulation and execution highlighted the complexities of crisis governance. The following section discusses these challenges in India's COVID-19 vaccination approach within the context of crisis management and policy response.

2.3 India's COVID-19 Vaccine Policy

2.3.1 The COVID-19 Vaccine

The COVID-19 vaccine emerged as the only effective way to save lives, and rapid and widespread vaccination was critical to end the pandemic. India, a global manufacturing hub and a major exporter of generic medicines, vaccines and other essential medical products, is hailed as the "pharmacy of the world".[47] For over a 1.3 billion population, India needed a domestically produced and indigenous vaccine[48] to meet its large demand more effectively and efficiently. There were serious expectations from India—both domestically and globally—that it would ramp up vaccine production, administer rapid inoculation in India and support equitable and swift access to COVID-19 vaccines globally. However, India did not fare well in its COVID-19 vaccine policy, with severe consequences at both domestic and global levels.

This section analyses the factors that led to a systemic failure in India's COVID-19 vaccine policy. India's vaccine policy has both technical and non-technical issues that need to be dealt with, including misinformation on vaccines, vaccine hesitancy, digital challenges, language and social barriers in vaccine roll-out, Aadhaar insistence, gender-related issues, barriers to access faced by senior citizens, people with special needs and Adivasis and forest dwellers and issues related to intellectual property rights and drugs regulation policy. However, this section is focused on five key issues related to investment in the research and development of vaccines: procurement orders, shortage of COVID-19 vaccine doses, vaccine pricing and India's vaccine diplomacy.

2.3.1.1 Funding Gaps: No Investment, No Aid, No Grants

On 19 April 2020, the Union Ministry of Health and Family Welfare (MoHFW) constituted a task force focused on COVID-19-related research and vaccine development.[49] Additionally, on 12 August 2020, a national expert group was instituted to conceptualise the administration, management and delivery mechanism for the COVID-19 vaccination.[50] However, no investment or were granted by the Union Government for the development and manufacture of COVID-19 vaccines. In an affidavit filed before the Supreme Court on 9 May 2021, the Government admitted that "no governmental aid, assistance or grant is made either for research or development of either Covaxin or Covishield".[51]

India's lack of preparedness in its COVID-19 vaccine policy was evident from the beginning. For instance, unlike the United States, the United Kingdom, the European Union and other countries, India did not invest in early vaccine research and development. This delay hindered the rapid development, procurement and mass distribution of the COVID-19 vaccines. Developed countries not only invested heavily in multiple vaccine candidates across the world but also placed advance procurement orders.[52] In contrast, the Union Government was caught in its *atmanirbhar Bharat* (self-reliant India) rhetoric and failed to act decisively to strategise a secure COVID-19 vaccine policy for the country. The Government both overestimated India's capacity to produce vaccines and underestimated the country's own vaccine need.[53] Without extending any support, it relied on local manufacturers to meet the country's demand and also to satisfy its "saviour of the world" complex.[54] The Government failed not only to invest in vaccine research and development and in expanding the country's vaccine manufacturing capacity but also to diversify India's vaccine sources, thus missing the critical period for placing orders for the vaccines.

2.3.1.2 *Delayed Procurement Order*

On 15 August 2020, from the Red Fort in Delhi, Prime Minister Narendra Modi announced India's roadmap for mass production and distribution of the COVID-19 vaccines.[55] On 28 December 2020, the MoHFW issued operational guidelines for the vaccine roll-out,[56] and on 3 January 2021, the Drugs Controller General of India officially approved the emergency use of two vaccines: Covishield by Serum Institute of India and Oxford AstraZeneca and Covaxin by Bharat Biotech. With this preparation, India was set to launch the "world's largest vaccination programme" on 16 January 2021,[57] prioritising vaccination for nurses, doctors and other frontline workers. However, the only thing missing was vaccine doses, for which the Union Government placed its first order on 11 January 2021—just five days before the commencement of the vaccination drive.[58]

India's COVID-19 vaccine policy fiasco began with its delayed purchase orders, leading to a slow start of the vaccination programme and contributing to the high human cost of COVID-19.[59] While many countries started signing advance procurement agreements and vaccine contracts as early as May 2020, the Union Government waited until January 2021 to place its first order.[60] Even then, the Government did not order sufficient doses. In January 2021, the Government ordered a measly 16.5 million vaccine doses for a population of 1.34 billion.[61] The next order, for 14.5 million doses, was placed on 10 February 2021.[62] The first substantial order of 120 million doses was finally placed on 21 March 2021,[63] around the time India was beginning to grapple with the second wave of COVID-19, India's worst catastrophe since Partition.[64]

2.3.1.3 *Vaccine Shortages*

One persistent problem since the beginning of India's COVID-19 vaccination programme was a shortage of vaccine doses. This scarcity hampered the vaccination programme to the point where inoculation was brought to a halt in several states.[65] Data show that the Union Government did not order enough doses for everyone.[66] As the outcry over the vaccine shortage grew, state governments ceaselessly reached out to the Union Government to address the inadequate supply and demanded transparency in vaccine policy decisions and interstate allocation processes.[67] Though the Government never acknowledged the shortage, it took several desperate remedial actions to address the vaccine shortage.

To begin with, on 17 March 2021, the Union Government constituted a six-member inter-ministerial panel to facilitate "capacity augmentation of domestic vaccines" manufactured for COVID-19.[68] In an unprecedented move in the last week of March 2021, the Government ordered the Serum Institute to halt the export of COVID-19 vaccines[69]—severely impacting the global vaccination programmes like the World Health Organisation's (WHO) COVID-19 Vaccine Global Access Facility (COVAX) initiative. Nevertheless, while people were struggling to find COVID-19 jabs during the unrelenting second wave of COVID-19, and the Government was exploring the possibilities of importing COVID-19 vaccines, Prime Minister Modi, on 8 April 2021, in a dramatic move, announced a *tika utsav* (vaccination festival) between 11 and 14 April 2021.[70]

Faced with an acute vaccine shortage and growing public outrage, the Government attempted to overturn its two irrational policy decisions. First, instead of depending solely on home-made vaccines, it began the process of importing foreign-made vaccines. Second, the Government turned back to revive and ramp up India's public vaccine manufacturers.

On 12 April 2021, the Union Government sanctioned fast-track emergency approval to foreign-made vaccines, provided they were prequalified by the WHO.[71] On 13 April 2021, the Government even approved Russia's Sputnik V vaccine,[72] which was not approved by the WHO. These vaccines were approved without waiting for the bridging trial results. However, these efforts failed, as none of these vaccines, except Sputnik V, reached India's vaccination centres. All this was a setback to India's long-standing position of being a global vaccine manufacturer and supplier and to the present Government's *atmanirbhar Bharat* rhetoric.

The failure of privately owned Bharat Biotech to deliver the vaccines as per orders, prompted the Union Government to go back to India's public vaccine manufacturers which were previously overlooked.[73] In April 2021, the government hastily roped in three public enterprises, namely Haffkine Bio-Pharmaceutical Corporation, Bharat Immunologicals and Biologicals Corporation and Indian Immunologicals Ltd, to produce Bharat Biotech's Covaxin.[74] However, these public enterprises were not in a state to produce and deliver the vaccines until 2022, given the complex and highly technical procedures involved. On 2 June 2021, Haffkine stated that it would take eight months to ramp up production,[75] while Bharat Immunologicals and Biologicals aimed to begin production by February 2022.[76] Therefore, amid the raging second wave, India's desperate wait to access vaccines only got longer.

Further, in another turn, on 19 April 2021, the Union Government—without any consultation with the state governments and against the advice of the National Technical Advisory Group on Immunisation[77]—announced a "Liberalised and Accelerated Phase 3 Strategy of COVID-19 Vaccination".[78] This new policy did three things: first, it shifted partial responsibility for vaccinating people aged 18–44 from the Union Government to state governments and private hospitals; second, it required India's vaccine suppliers to supply 50 per cent of its production to the Union Government and the remaining equally to the state governments and private hospitals; and thirdly, it allowed vaccine manufacturers to decide differential pricing for their supplies to state governments and private hospitals.[79]

This was the disastrous attempt by the Union Government to evade its obligation to vaccinate people and its responsibility for the vaccine shortage. Under the constitutional scheme, the Union Government has considerable powers through fiscal control, which traditionally translated into centralised planning and policy-making with decentralised implementation and distribution.[80] However, the Government's attempt to reverse India's long-standing universal vaccination policy[81] through the liberalised vaccine policy brought the debate around COVID-19 vaccine pricing before the Supreme Court of India.

2.3.1.4 Vaccine Pricing

In January 2020, India's COVID-19 vaccination programme started with free vaccination for all healthcare workers and frontline workers at government-run facilities. However, in the second phase of the vaccination programme, which began on 1 March 2021, the Union Government allowed private entities to deliver paid COVID-19 inoculation at a prescribed rate. While most countries provided free universal vaccination, the Union Government's decision to involve private entities led to deregulation of procurement and vaccine pricing, fragmentation of India's vaccine market[82] and prevention of universal access to vaccination.

This can be understood by comparing the vaccine procurement prices before and after the Government announced the liberalised vaccine policy, effective from 1 May 2021.

Initially, as per the Parliamentary Standing Committee Report, the Serum Institute of India quoted a price of ₹250 per dose of Covishield, which the Union Government negotiated to ₹200 per dose. Bharat Biotech quoted a price of ₹350 per dose of Covaxin, which finally came to ₹206 per dose after Bharat Biotech offered 30 per cent doses free of cost.[83] Nevertheless, the Union Government maintained before the Supreme Court that it was procuring both the vaccines at the rate of ₹150 per dose.[84] On 27 Feb 2021, the Government capped the vaccine price at ₹250 per dose for private hospitals, including hospital's administration fee.[85]

After the announcement of liberalised vaccine policy, prices went up for state governments and private hospitals. Serum Institute offered Covishield to state governments at ₹400 and to private hospitals at ₹600 per dose.[86] Bharat Biotech offered Covaxin to state governments at ₹600 per dose and to private hospitals at ₹1,200 per dose.[87] Russia's Sputnik V vaccine was priced at ₹948 plus a 5 per cent Goods and Services Tax.[88] Both Serum Institute and Bharat Biotech maintained the rate of ₹150 per dose for the Union Government.

The Supreme Court reviewed several petitions related to India's COVID-19 vaccine policy,[89] focusing on various aspects of the right to health vis-à-vis access to life-saving medicines. The most prominent was the court's sou motu motion, in which it examined the issues related to vaccine availability and access, procurement policy and vaccine mandate.[90] On 27 April 2021, the Supreme Court pulled up the Union Government and expressed concerns regarding the different prices for vaccines.[91] The court directed the Government to clarify detailed questions on the vaccine policy, including "the basis and rationale which has been adopted by the Union Government in regard to the pricing of the vaccine".[92] Following the Supreme Court's intervention, Covishield reduced the price for state governments from ₹400 to ₹300[93] and Covaxin slashed the price for state governments from ₹600 to ₹400 per dose.[94] However, the price drop did not aid either the Union Government or the vaccine manufacturers. The apex court on 31 May 2021, in a detailed order, ruled that the Union Government's liberalised policy is "prima facie arbitrary and irrational"[95] and warned the Government that paid vaccination "could have serious implication[s] on the fundamental [Article 14] right to equality and [Article 21] the right to health of persons".[96]

After the Supreme Court reprimanded the Union Government, the Government decided to partially retract the liberalised policy. On 7 June 2021, Prime Minister Modi himself announced[97] that the Union Government would procure the state government's vaccine share of 25 per cent, taking the Union Government's procurement to 75 per cent. However, the remaining 25 per cent share of vaccines was left for private entities at a capped price of ₹780, ₹1,410 and ₹1,145 per dose for Covishield, Covaxin and Sputnik V, respectively[98] (as of 8 June 2021). In July 2022, the Union Government revised the vaccine price to ₹215 for Covishield and ₹225 for Covaxin.[99]

2.3.1.5 "Vaccine Maitri": Export Missteps

On 20 January 2021, India launched its global vaccine assistance programme under the *Vaccine Maitri* (vaccine friendship) initiative[100] to fulfil its commitment to global vaccine equity.[101] The Union Government began shipping vaccines to the world, with Prime Minister Modi asserting at the 2021 World Economic Forum that "India is saving the lives of people in many other countries of the world by sending COVID vaccines"[102]; the MoFHW stated that India had beaten the COVID-19 pandemic.[103] As per the data published by the Union Ministry of External Affairs,[104] starting from January 2021, India exported 66.4 million doses of Covishield and Covaxin either as a gift or under commercial contracts, or WHO's COVAX, until the Government put an embargo on vaccine exports in April 2021.[105] It is pertinent to note that by the time India put restrictions on export, it had already shipped more vaccine doses than it had administered to its own people.[106] For instance, by the time India restricted vaccine export, it had already exported 66 million doses to 95 countries[107] while administering 52 million doses to its own population.[108]

India's hasty decision to export vaccines for diplomatic gains delayed access for India's vulnerable population's access to vaccines and it put further strain on the Serum Institute to deliver on contractual obligations.[109] Within two months, India went from being a vaccine exporter to looking for possibilities to import vaccines.[110] The Government's poor planning and failure to estimate India's own vaccination needs caused an acute vaccine shortage during the remorseless second wave. Faced with public fury and criticism from the judiciary,[111] the Union Government, without any formal declaration, directed the Serum Institute to halt vaccine exports, causing severe constraints to the WHO's COVAX initiative.

The Serum Institute had received a license to produce Oxford-AstraZeneca's Covishield under an agreement to supply 200 million vaccine doses to low-income countries, including India and its neighbours Bangladesh, Nepal and Sri Lanka,[112] under the COVAX initiative.[113] However, the de facto export ban disrupted vaccine supplies to countries dependent on COVAX, prolonging the pandemic. This decision to restrict vaccine export during the second wave dented India's vaccine altruism image and its perception as a reliable vaccine supplier.[114] In October 2021, six months after the export ban on vaccines, India resumed the *Vaccine Maitri* initiative.[115]

Vaccination was the safest and most strategic option to end the pandemic, making a case for the human right to access essential medicines vis-à-vis vaccines even stronger. The courts have repeatedly reiterated the State's obligation to guarantee people's access to life-saving medicines and drugs. The above review demonstrates the facts related to India's vaccine policy decisions and exposes the Government's failure to ensure effective and free universal access to the COVID-19 vaccine. One of the many reasons for this failure is the absence of a clear legislative framework on the right to healthcare, which defines justiciable rights and duties related to healthcare and medicines and provides a clear directive on the State's response to a public health emergency like COVID-19 pandemic. In framing the response to the COVID-19 pandemic, the Government neglected the court's directives related to the right to access medicines.

2.4 The Right to Health

Health is a universally recognised human right,[116] inextricably linked to the overall human condition,[117] development[118] and social empowerment of individuals.[119] It is key to human dignity and the enjoyment of all other human rights.[120] Despite these imperatives, the right to health is not recognised as a legal right in India. Since Independence, India has progressed in medical sciences and research, but on the ground, it has failed to provide access to affordable, equitable and quality healthcare to its 1.3 billion population. The COVID-19 pandemic has exposed and aggravated India's frail healthcare system, which has struggled due to low public health expenditure and the lack of a statutory framework that guarantees and binds the State to respect, protect and fulfil the human right to health.[121]

While the Indian Constitution does not provide a right to health or healthcare, it provides diluted provisions on public health in the form of DPSPs in Part IV of the Constitution. On the subject of health, the DPSPs under Article 39 (e) and (f) outline the State's obligations to secure the health of workers and children; Article 42 requires the State to provide just and humane conditions of work and maternity relief; and Article 47 casts the duty on the State to raise the nutrition levels, improve living standards and enhance public health.

Over the last seven decades, the DPSPs have been extensively interpreted and justified by incorporating the underlying objectives of fundamental rights. The Supreme Court has defined the DPSPs as social goals[122] and ruled that fundamental rights and directive principles are complementary and supplementary to each other.[123] In *Bandhua Mukti Morcha v. Union of India and others*,[124] the court has linked the directive principles related to health/public health with the fundamental right to life, to interpret the right to health under the Constitution. Justice Bhagwati observed: "This right to live with human dignity enshrined in Article 21 derives its life breath from the Directive Principles of State Policy and particularly clauses (e) and (f) of Article 39 and Article 41 and 42."[125] Constitutional principles on social security, a decent standard of living and adequate public services form the basis of the right to health and healthcare.[126] However, the only constitutional and legal constraint in translating the constitutional norm to promote health into a legal right is the principle of justiciability,[127] which can only be achieved through legislation enacted by the Parliament.

The courts have interpreted the right to health under Article 21 in two broad aspects: the right to access medicines/medical facilities and the right to a healthy life,[128] and touched multiple aspects of health—access to emergency medical care, access to medicines and treatment, health care financing, non-discrimination in access to healthcare, the health of women and children, environmental protection to ensure overall health and even access to COVID-19 vaccines.[129] While the jurisprudence developed by the courts has significantly contributed to building a framework on the right to health, the judiciary has been reluctant to hold the government accountable for its failure to fulfil its statutory obligations[130] towards public health. Nevertheless, this case-law-based framework has substantial implications, especially in the absence of a legislative framework which guarantees and protects the right to health and defines the State's role and duties to formulate public health policies to prevent the spread of infectious diseases and respond to pandemics while maintaining and respecting human rights.

2.5 Consequences of Failure

The judiciary has constructed an elaborated jurisprudence on the right to health. Although the courts have not engaged with the larger inter-sectional issues[131] within the right to health, they have established a rights-based socio-economic jurisprudence on health. In the absence of a legislative framework that guarantees and protects the rights related to health, this socio-economic jurisprudence presents a blue-print for a framework on the right to health. The absence of a coherent legislative and policy framework, coupled with economic constraints, has resulted in a fragmented and dysfunctional healthcare system in India. While the COVID-19 pandemic did not cause the disjointed state of India's public health system, it has uncovered the deep-rooted issues of socio-economic inequalities in access, availability and affordability of healthcare. Furthermore, the pandemic has also exposed the State's negligence towards public health, which is noticeable in India's COVID-19 vaccine policy.

This survey of India's vaccine policy demonstrates the Union Government's complacency in effectively procuring and distributing the COVID-19 vaccines. While failing to consider the judicial framework on the right to health, the Government has dealt with the pandemic through executive decrees and policy provisions. The inconsistent policy responses prolonged the pandemic, resulting in severe economic damage[132] and tragic human costs.[133] For instance, during the second wave of the COVID-19 pandemic, the seven-day average of cases surged from about 16,000 in March 2021 to nearly 4,00,000 in May 2021.[134] Daily reported deaths exceeded 4,000 on 26 May 2021,[135] contributing to an estimated 4.7 million deaths during 2020–2021, according to the WHO.[136] The sudden shock of the pandemic brought economic activities to a standstill,[137] causing India's GDP to slump by 23.9 per cent.[138] In the receding economy, the lives and livelihoods of marginal social groups spiralled down further, and there was limited recovery post-pandemic. Less-educated workers, who were engaged in low-paying jobs within the informal sector,[139] were severely affected by the loss of livelihood, reduced access to essential services and lack of social security, pushing millions into poverty.[140]

During an emergency, citizens in a democracy may relinquish some of their fundamental rights in favour of the State so that the State can act on behalf of the citizens to address the challenges posed by such an emergency and protect their rights from inevitable dangers. The Government's response to the pandemic was top-down authoritarian, and several fundamental rights of the citizens were compromised in the process. Yet, the Indian government failed to fulfil its moral obligation and constitutional duty to protect people's fundamental right to life.

Notes

1 Vani K. Borooach, Inequality in health outcomes in India: The role of caste and religion, in Sukhdeo Thorat and Katherine S Newman (eds.), *Blocked by Caste—Economic Discrimination in Modern India*, New Delhi: Oxford University Press, 2010: 179–80.

2 Vani K. Borooach, *Global Spending on Health: Weathering the Storm*, Geneva: World Health Organization, 2020: 67. www.who.int/publications/i/item/9789240017788.

3 Longjam Dineshwori, Maternal and newborn deaths: What India is doing to address the issue and what more can be done?, *The HealthSite*, 19 January 2023. www.thehealthsite.com/pregnancy/maternal-and-newborn-deaths-what-india-is-doing-to-address-the-issue-and-what-more-can-be-done-945674/.
4 Sounak Mukhopadhyay, India's life expectancy to hit 82 by 2100, as per UN estimates, *LiveMint*, 9 October 2022. www.livemint.com/news/india/indias-life-expectancy-to-hit-82-by-2100-as-per-un-estimates-11665298822775.html.
5 UNDP, *Human Development Report 2023–24: Breaking the Gridlock—Reimagining Cooperation in a Polarized World*, New York: UNDP, 2024. https://hdr.undp.org/system/files/documents/global-report-document/hdr2023-24reporten.pdf.
6 7th Schedule (Article 246) of the Constitution of India.
7 Ravi Duggal, Health and development in India: Moving towards the right to health, in José M. Zuniga, Stephen P. Marks, and Lawrence O. Gostin (eds.), *Advancing the Human Right to Health*, Oxford: Oxford University Press, 2013: 118–19.
8 Act No. 53 of 2005.
9 Maitreyi Gupta, Indian government fails to protect right to life and health in second wave of Covid-19 pandemic, *International Commission of Jurist*, 29 April 2021. www.icj.org/indian-government-fails-to-protect-right-to-life-and-health-in-second-wave-of-covid-19-pandemic/.
10 Jayati Ghosh, *The Making of a Catastrophe: The Disastrous Economic Fallout of the COVID-19 Pandemic in India*, New Delhi: Aleph Book Company, 2022: viii–xiii.
11 Vidya Krishnan, and Sarah Nabia, The Indian government used the pandemic to craft a political image and failed to save lives, *The Caravan*, 14 September 2021. https://caravanmagazine.in/health/the-indian-government-used-the-pandemic-to-craft-a-political-image.
12 Nikita Kansal, Covid-19 hitting India's poor the hardest, *East Asia Forum*, 18 May 2021. https://eastasiaforum.org/2021/05/18/covid-19-hitting-indias-poor-the-hardest/.
13 *Atul Kumar Sharma v. Govt of N.C.T. of Delhi & Ors.* W.P. (C) 5096/2021.
14 "We have failed": Delhi HC's Anguish over inability to help secure ICU bed after petitioner passes away, *The Leaflet: Constitution First*, 1 May 2021. https://theleaflet.in/we-have-failed-delhi-hcs-anguish-over-inability-to-help-secure-icu-bed-after-petitioner-passes-away-state-failed-to-protect-a-persons-right-to-life-it-says/.
15 India's National Government Looks Increasingly Hapless, *The Economist*, 8 May 2021. www.economist.com/asia/2021/05/08/indias-national-government-looks-increasingly-hapless.
16 Vikas Pandey, India Covid: Delhi hospitals pleas for oxygen as more patients Dia, *BBC*, 3 May 2021. www.bbc.com/news/world-asia-india-56940595.
17 Vikas Pandey, Frames of crematorium furnaces melt due to rush of bodies in Gujarat, *Hindustan Times*, 13 April 2021. www.hindustantimes.com/india-news/covid19-frames-of-crematorium-furnaces-melt-due-to-rush-of-bodies-in-gujarat-101618306897681.html.
18 Geeta Pandey, India's holiest river, the Ganges, has been swollen with bodies in recent days, *BBC*, 19 May 2021. www.bbc.com/news/world-asia-india-57154564.
19 Richard Horton, *The COVID-19 Catastrophe: What's Gone Wrong and How to Stop It Happening Again*, Cambridge: Polity Press, 2021: 67.
20 Richard Horton, *Healthy States Progressive India: Report on the Ranks of States and Union Territories*, New Delhi: NITI Aayog, 2019. http://social.niti.gov.in/uploads/sample/health_index_report.pdf.
21 Manish Tewari, India's fight against health emergencies: In search of a legal architecture, *ORF Issue Brief*, 31 March 2020. www.orfonline.org/research/

indias-fight-against-health-emergencies-in-search-of-a-legal-architecture-63884/#_edn16.

22 Fran M. Snowden, *Epidemics and Society: From the Black Death to the Present*. New Haven, CT: Yale University Press, 2019.

23 Kaleeswaram Raj, Freedom in the time of COVID-19, in Kaleeswaram Raj (ed.), *Constitutional Concerns: Writings on Law and Life*, New Delhi: Tulika Books, 2022: 83.

24 Act No. 3 of 1897.

25 Kim D'Souza, Drafting a public health emergency preparedness and response law, towards a post-Covid India: 25 governance challenges and legal reforms, *Vidhi Centre for Legal Policy*, 24 July 2020: 4–6. https://vidhilegalpolicy.in/wp-content/uploads/2020/07/Towards-A-Post-Covid-India_Vidhi-Centre-for-Legal-Policy.pdf.

26 Gautam Bhatia, India: Covid-19, the executive, and the judiciary, *OpinioJuris*, 26 July 2021. https://opiniojuris.org/2021/07/26/covid-19-and-courts-symposium-india-covid-19-the-executive-and-the-judiciary/.

27 Gautam Bhatia, India: Covid-19, the executive, and the judiciary, *OpinioJuris*, 26 July 2021. https://opiniojuris.org/2021/07/26/covid-19-and-courts-symposium-india-covid-19-the-executive-and-the-judiciary/.

28 Gautam Bhatia, Government of India issues orders prescribing lockdown for containment of Covid-19 epidemic in the country, *Press Information Bureau*, 24 March 2020. www.mha.gov.in/sites/default/files/PR_NationalLockdown_26032020_0.pdf.

29 Jeffrey Gettleman, and Kai Schultz, Modi orders 3-week total lockdown for all 1.3 billion Indians, *The New York Times*, 24 March 2020. www.nytimes.com/2020/03/24/world/asia/india-coronavirus-lockdown.html.

30 Nikhil Pratap, and Kashish Aneja, 1.3 billion people. One virus. How much privacy?, *The Wire*, 30 March 2020. https://thewire.in/government/covid-19-pandemic-privacy-india.

31 Billy Perrigo, The India government is silencing critics even as its Covid-19 crisis surges, *Time*, 29 April 2021. https://time.com/6005847/india-government-silencing-critics-covid-19/.

32 Kaleeswaram Raj, Governance during the pandemic, in Kaleeswaram Raj (ed.), *Constitutional Concerns: Writings on Law and Life*, New Delhi: Tulika Books, 2022: 130–31.

33 The Wire Staff, Religious, political mass gatherings contributed to Covid-19 resurgence in India: WHO, *The Wire*, 13 May 2021. https://thewire.in/health/religious-political-mass-gatherings-contributed-to-covid-19-resurgence-in-india-who.

34 Preamble to the Constitution of India.

35 Gopal Subramanium, Emergency provisions under the Indian Constitution, in B. N. Kripal, Ashok H. Desai, and Gopal Subramanium et al. (eds.), *Supreme but Not Infallible: Essays in Honour of the Supreme Court of India*, New Delhi: Oxford University Press, 2004: 134.

36 n. 32 *Kaleeswaram*: 133.

37 *Mahabir Auto Service v. Indian Oil Corporations* (1990) 3 SCC 752.

38 Leela Simon, and Chiranjivi J. Nirmal, Fundamental rights: The constitutional context of human rights, in Chiranjivi J. Nirmal (ed.), *Human Rights in India: Historical, Social and Political Perspective*, New Delhi: Oxford University Press, 2004: 43.

39 *Kesavananda Bharti v. State of Kerala* (1973) 1 SCC J 17.

40 Article 359 of the Constitution of India;—*The Constitution (Forty-Constitutional Amendment) Act, 1978*, New Delhi: Ministry of Law, Justice and Company Affairs, Government of India, 1978.

41 *Maneka Gandhi v. Union of India* AIR 1978 SC 27.
42 Article 352 of the Constitution of India.
43 n. 26 *Bhatia*.
44 *Emergency Measures and COVID-19 Guidance*, Geneva: OHCHR, 27 April 2020. www.ohchr.org/sites/default/files/Documents/Events/EmergencyMeasures_COVID19.pdf.
45 Indira Jaising, Constitution and courts in India, *The Leaflet: Constitution First*, 5 April 2020. https://theleaflet.in/constitution-and-courts-in-the-time-of-corona/.
46 n. 35 *Subramanium*: 151.
47 Nikhil S. Masurkar, Why is India the pharmacy of the world?, *Financial Express*, 25 September 2021. www.financialexpress.com/lifestyle/health/why-is-india-the-pharmacy-of-the-world/2337554/.
48 Chandrakant Lahariya, Gangandeep Kang, and Randeep Guleria, *Till We Win: India's Fight Against the COVID-19 Pandemic*, New Delhi: Penguin Book, 2020: 188.
49 Chandrakant Lahariya, A high-level task force, co-chaired by member, NITI AAYOG and principal scientific adviser, formed to enable Covid-19 related research and vaccine development: Health ministry, *Press Information Bureau*, 19 April 2020. https://pib.gov.in/Pressreleaseshare.aspx?PRID=1616154.
50 Chandrakant Lahariya, National expert group on vaccine administration for Covid-19 deliberates on strategy to ensure Covid-19 vaccines' availability and its delivery mechanism, *Press Information Bureau*, 12 August 2020. https://pib.gov.in/PressReleasePage.aspx?PRID=1645363.
51 *In Re: Distribution of Essential Supplies and Services During Pandemic*. Sou Moto Writ Petition (C) No. 3/2021. Affidavit dated 09.05.2021 on behalf of the Union of India: 55–56. www.livelaw.in/pdf_upload/uoi-affidavit-9052021-final-with-annexures-1–91–393168.pdf.
52 Rakesh Sood, Kriti Kapur, and Oommen C. Kurian, *India's Vaccine Rollout: A Reality Check* (ORF Special Report No. 139), New Delhi: Observer Research Foundation, 2021: 11. https://orfonline.org/wp-content/uploads/2021/05/ORF_SpecialReport_139_Vaccination_FinalForUpload.pdf.
53 Neeta Sanghi, How the Modi government overestimated India's capacity to make Covid-19 vaccines, *The Wire Science*, 22 April 2021. https://science.thewire.in/health/narendra-modi-government-overestimated-india-covid-vaccine-manufacturing-capacity-shortage/.
54 Neeta Sanghi, How the Modi government overestimated India's capacity to make Covid-19 vaccines, *The Wire Science*, 22 April 2021. https://science.thewire.in/health/narendra-modi-government-overestimated-india-covid-vaccine-manufacturing-capacity-shortage/.
55 Neeta Sanghi, 3 Covid-19 vaccines being tested, plan ready for mass distribution: PM Modi, *The Times of India*, 15 August 2020. https://timesofindia.indiatimes.com/india/pm-modi-says-india-set-to-mass-produce-covid-19-vaccine-launches-health-mission/articleshow/77558341.cms.
56 Neeta Sanghi, *COVID-19 Vaccine. Operational Guidelines*, New Delhi: Ministry of Health and Family Welfare, Government of India, 2020. www.mohfw.gov.in/pdf/COVID19VaccineOG111Chapter16.pdf.
57 Neeta Sanghi, *Precautions and Contraindications of COVID-19 Vaccination*, New Delhi: Ministry of Health and Family Welfare, Government of India, 2021. www.mohfw.gov.in/pdf/LetterfromAddlSecyMoHFWregContraindicationsandFactsheetforCOVID19vaccines.PDF.
58 V. Shridhar, Covid-19: Vaccine follies, *Frontline*, 1 June 2021. https://frontline.thehindu.com/covid-19/covid19-vaccine-follies-india-vaccine-story-missteps-by-narendra-modi-led-bjp-government/article34689540.ece.

59 Oommen C. Kurian, COVID-19 pandemic response: Comparing the Indian and Chinese approaches, *Expert Speak—Observer Research Foundation*, 20 September 2021. https://www.orfonline.org/expert-speak/covid-19-pandemic-response-comparing-the-indian-and-chinese-approaches/.

60 G. S. Mudur, How India landed in Covid vaccine mess, *The Telegraph*, 19 April 2021. www.telegraphindia.com/india/how-we-landed-in-covid-vaccine-mess/cid/1812969?utm_source=twitter&utm_medium=social&utm_campaign=tt_daily_twit.

61 Prasanna Mohanty, *An Unkept Promise: What Derailed the Indian Economy*, New Delhi: Sage, 2022: 131.

62 Rhythma Kaul, Govt orders 14.5mn more doses as preparation for second dose begin, *Hindustan Times*, 10 February 2021. www.hindustantimes.com/india-news/covid19-govt-orders-14-5mn-more-doses-as-preparation-for-second-dose-begins-101612911222590.html.

63 Anonna Dutt, 120 million doses ordered as vaccine urgency deepens, *Hindustan Times*, 21 March 2021. www.hindustantimes.com/india-news/120mn-doses-ordered-as-vaccine-urgency-deepens-101616264676262.html.

64 The Lancet COVID-19 Commission: India Task Force, Managing India's Second COVID-19 Wave: Urgent Steps, *The Lancet*, 2021. https://static1.squarespace.com/static/5ef3652ab722df11fcb2ba5d/t/6076f57d3b43fb2db4a7c9c9/1618408831746/India+TF+Policy+Brief+April+2021.pdf.

65 The Lancet COVID-19 Commission: India Task Force, 10 States face severe Covid-19 vaccine shortage. Here's is a list, *Hindustan Times*, 10 April 2021. www.hindustantimes.com/india-news/10-states-face-severe-covid-19-vaccine-shortage-here-s-a-list-101618047783891.html.

66 Shreya Raman, and Kriti Kapur, India may not have enough doses to meet its Covid vaccination targets, data show, *IndiaSpend*, 13 April 2021. www.indiaspend.com/covid-19/india-may-not-have-enough-doses-to-meet-its-covid-vaccination-targets-data-show-741382.

67 Manasi Phadke, Himani Chandna, and Aneesha Bedi, Modi govt says there's no vaccine shortage, but states and hospitals tell a different story, *The Print*, 8 April 2021. https://theprint.in/health/modi-govt-says-theres-no-vaccine-shortage-but-states-hospitals-tell-a-different-story/636054/.

68 Stephanie Findlay, Michael Peel, and Donato Paolo Mancini, India blocks vaccine exports in blow to dozens of nations, *Financial Times*, 25 March 2021. www.ft.com/content/5349389c-8313-41e0-9a67-58274e24a019.

69 n. 53 *Sanghi*.

70 In PM Modi's CMs meet, vaccine shortage takes centre stage, *The Wire Science*, 9 April 2021. https://science.thewire.in/health/covid-19-in-pm-modis-cms-meet-vaccine-shortage-takes-centre-stage/.

71 India to fast-track approvals for foreign-produced Covid-19 vaccines, *The Wire Science*, 13 April 2021. https://science.thewire.in/health/india-fast-tracks-emergency-approvals-for-foreign-produced-covid-19-vaccines/.

72 Niham Prusty, and Krishna N. Das, Drug controller general of India approves Russia's Sputnik V vaccine, *The Wire Science*, 13 April 2021. https://science.thewire.in/health/covid-19-drug-controller-general-of-india-approves-russias-sputnik-v-vaccine/.

73 Swagata Yadavar, India's bumbling vaccine policy: How India failed to ensure just and equitable access to vaccines for its population at every step, in Yogesh Jain and Sarah Nabia (eds.), *COVID-19—A View From the Margin*, New Delhi: Manohar, 2022: 351.

74 Swagata Yadavar, India readies state-run firms to manufacture Covaxin, *Live Mint*, 16 May 2021. www.livemint.com/news/india/india-readies-state-run-firms-to-manufacture-covaxin-11621078961652.html.

75 Leroy Leo, Haffkine to produce 228 million doses of Covaxin annually at Mumbai facility, *Live Mint*, 2 June 2021. www.livemint.com/companies/news/haffkine-to-produce-228-million-doses-of-covaxin-annually-at-mumbai-facility/amp-11622630498319.html.

76 Teena Thacker, State BIBCOL set begin production of Bharat Bio's Covaxin by February 2022, *Economics Times*, 28 July 2021. https://m.economictimes.com/industry/healthcare/biotech/state-owned-bibcol-set-to-begin-production-of-bharat-bios-covaxin-by-february-2022/amp_articleshow/84814057.cms.

77 n. 61 *Mohanty*: 133–34.

78 Ministry of Health and Family Welfare. Government of India. Government announces a liberalised and accelerated Phase 3 strategy of Covid-19 vaccination from 1st May, *Press Information Bureau*, 19 April 2021. https://pib.gov.in/PressReleasePage.aspx?PRID=1712710.

79 Ministry of Health and Family Welfare. Government of India. Government announces a liberalised and accelerated Phase 3 strategy of Covid-19 vaccination from 1st May. *Press Information Bureau*, 19 April 2021. https://pib.gov.in/PressReleasePage.aspx?PRID=1712710.

80 Monica Das Gupta, and Manju Rani, *India's Public Health System: How Well Does It Function at the National Level? (Policy Research Working Paper 3447)*, Washington, DC: World Bank, 2004: 3. https://openknowledge.worldbank.org/bitstream/handle/10986/14215/WPS3447.pdf?sequence=1&tnqh_x0026;isAllowed=y.

81 R. Ramakumar, Politics and economics of vaccine policy, *Economic & Politically Weekly* 56 (18) (2021): 8.

82 R. Ramakumar, India's 'arbitrary and irrational' vaccine policy spells trouble, *East Asia Forum*, 27 July 2021. www.eastasiaforum.org/2021/07/27/indias-arbitrary-and-irrational-vaccine-policy-spells-trouble/.

83 Parliamentary Standing Committee on Health and Family Welfare, *One Hundred Thirty Seventh Report on Vaccine Development, Distribution Management and Mitigation of Pandemic COVID-19*, New Delhi: Rajya Sabha Secretariat, 2022: 35.

84 *In Re: Distribution of Essential Supplies and Services During Pandemic*, Sou Moto Writ (Civil) No. 3/2021, Order dated 31 May 2021: 7. https://main.sci.gov.in/supremecourt/2021/11001/11001_2021_35_301_28040_Judgement_31-May-2021.pdf.

85 Nisha Nambiar, and Sushmi Dey, Covid vaccine price to be capped at Rs 250 per dose at private hospitals, *Times of India*, 28 February 2021. https://timesofindia.indiatimes.com/india/covid-vax-price-to-be-capped-at-r250/dose-at-private-hospitals/articleshow/81250696.cms.

86 The Wire Staff, Coviedshield will be Rs 400 for state govts, Rs 600 in private hospitals: Serum Institute, *The Wire*, 21 April 2021. https://science.thewire.in/health/covishield-rs-400-state-govternments-rs-600-private-hospitals-serum-institute-announcement/.

87 The Wire Staff, Everything you wanted to know about the price of vaccines in India, *The Wire*, 26 April 2021. https://thewire.in/government/everything-you-wanted-to-know-about-the-price-of-vaccines-in-india.

88 The Wire Staff, Russia's Sputnik V Vaccine for covid priced at Rs 948 plus 5% GST in India, *Business Standard*, 14 May 2021. www.business-standard.com/article/current-affairs/russia-s-sputnik-v-vaccine-for-covid-priced-at-rs-948-in-india-dr-reddy-s-121051400460_1.html.

89 *Jacob Puliyel v Union of India* (2022) SCC OnLine SC 533; and *Rachna Gangu v Union of India* (2022) SCC OnLine SC 1125.

90 *In Re: Distribution of Essential Supplies and Services During Pandemic* (2021) 7 SCC 772.

91 "Different manufacturers coming with different prices": Supreme Court asks centre to explain rationale of Covid vaccine pricing, *Live Law*, 27 April 2021. www.livelaw.in/top-stories/supreme-court-asks-centre-to-explain-rationale-of-covid-vaccine-pricing-173205.

92 *In Re: Distribution of Essential Supplies and Services During Pandemic*. Sou Moto Writ Petition (C) No. 3/2021, Order dated 27 April 2021. www.livelaw.in/pdf_upload/92-11001202135302277800rder27-apr-2021-392537.pdf.
93 Shoumojit Banerjee, Serum Institute of India cuts Covishield vaccine price for States to Rs 300 per dose, *The Hindu*, 28 April 2021. www.thehindu.com/news/national/serum-institute-of-india-cuts-covishield-vaccine-price-for-states-to-300-per-dose/article34431403.ece.
94 Shoumojit Banerjee, Bharat Biotech cuts Covaxin price to Rs 400 per dose for States, *Business Today*, 29 April 2021. www.businesstoday.in/latest/economy-politics/story/breaking-bharat-biotech-cuts-covaxin-price-to-rs-400-per-dose-for-states-294627-2021-04-29.
95 n. 92 *In Re: Distribution*: 18.
96 n. 92 *In Re: Distribution*: 30.
97 Divya Chandra, Govt changed vaccine policy before SC order? Here are the facts, *The Quint*, 8 June 2021. www.thequint.com/coronavirus/did-government-change-vaccination-policy-before-supreme-court-order-timeline#read-more.
98 Aparna Banerjee, Centre releases revised prices of Covishield, Covaxin, Sputnik jabs for Pvt hospitals, *Live Mint*, 8 June 2021. www.livemint.com/news/india/centre-releases-revised-prices-of-covishield-covaxin-sputnik-jabs-for-pvt-hospitals-check-details-11623166137696.html.
99 Abantika Ghosh, Modi govt finally raises vaccine prices, will pay Rs 215 for Covishield, Rs 225 for Covaxin, *The Print*, 16 July 2021. https://theprint.in/health/modi-govt-finally-raises-vaccine-prices-will-pay-rs-215-for-covishield-rs-225-for-covaxin/696852/.
100 Devika Chawla, Diplomacy in difficult times: India's "Vaccine Maitri" initiative, *Invest India*, 31 March 2021. www.investindia.gov.in/team-india-blogs/diplomacy-difficult-times-indias-vaccine-maitri-initiative.
101 Jyoti Sharma, and S. K. Varshney, 'India's vaccine diplomacy aids global access to Covid-19 jabs, *Nature India*, 17 February 2021. www.nature.com/articles/nindia.2021.31.
102 Aparna Banerjee, Modi at World Economic Forum: Many more COVID vaccines will come from India, say PM, *Live Mint*, 28 January 2021. www.livemint.com/news/india/wef-live-updates-many-more-covid-vaccines-will-come-from-india-s ays-pm-modi-11611836042629.html.
103 Salil Ahuja, In their own words: How India's leaders mishandled the Covid crisis, *News laundry*, 30 April 2021. www.newslaundry.com/2021/04/30/in-their-own-words-how-indias-leaders-mishandled-the-covid-crisis.
104 Ministry of External Affairs, Vaccine supply. *Government of India*. www.mea.gov.in/vaccine-supply.htm.
105 Ministry of External Affairs, India temporarily halts Oxford-AstraZeneca vaccine exports, *BBC*, 24 March 2021. www.bbc.com/news/world-asia-india-56513371.
106 Jeffrey Gettleman, Schmall Emily, and Mujib Mashal, India cuts back on vaccine exports as infections surge at home, *The New York Times*, 25 March 2021. www.nytimes.com/2021/03/25/world/asia/india-covid-vaccine-astrazeneca.html.
107 n. 104 *Ministry of External Affairs*.
108 Amitabh Kant, One billion doses: India's leadership in the world, *Niti Ayog*, 20 October 2021, www.niti.gov.in/one-billion-doses-indias-leadership-world#:~:text=Before%20pausing%20exports%20owing%20to,Myanmar%2C%20Bangladesh%2C%20and%20Iran; and Edouard Mathieu, Hannah Ritchie, and Lucas Rodés-Guirao et al., India: Coronavirus pandemic country profile—vaccination, *Our World in Data*, 2024. https://ourworldindata.org/coronavirus/country/india.

109 Manoj Joshi, India's gains from 'vaccine diplomacy'—if any—will be small, transient and pyrrhic, *The Wire*, 24 January 2021. https://thewire.in/diplomacy/india-vaccine-exports-diplomacy-brazil-china.
110 Manavi Kapur, In a span of one month, India has gone from shipping out Covid-19 aid to receiving it, *Quartz*, 5 May 2021. https://qz.com/india/2004268/india-went-from-sending-vaccines-to-receiving-foreign-covid-aid.
111 Manavi Kapur, It's a shame that while government knew of magnitude of Covid second wave, it never planned things in advance: Allahabad High Court', *LiveLaw*, 19 April 2021. www.livelaw.in/top-stories/allahabad-high-court-uttar-pradesh-lockdown-covid19-second-wave-govt-didnt-plan-172810.
112 Richa Chintan, How India and Covax failed the South Asian countries, *News-Click*, 24 June 2021. www.newsclick.in/COVID-19-India-COVAX-failed-South-Asian-Countries.
113 Emily Schmall, and Karan Deep Singh, India and its vaccine maker stumble over their pandemic promises, *The New York Times*, 7 May 2021. www.nytimes.com/2021/05/07/world/india-serum-institute-covid19.html?action=click&module=RelatedLinks&pgtype=Article.
114 Devirupa Mitra, With none of the earlier fanfare in sight, India resumes Covid-19 vaccine export, *The Wire*, 27 November 2021. https://thewire.in/diplomacy/india-covid-19-vaccine-maitri-branding.
115 Devirupa Mitra, India resumed Covid-19 vaccine export, *The Hindu*, 14 October 2021. www.thehindu.com/news/national/india-resumes-covid-19-vaccine-export/article36999436.ece.
116 Article 5 (e) (iv), International Convention on the Elimination of All Forms of Racial Discrimination, 1965; Article 12, International Covenant on Economic, Social and Cultural Rights, 1966; Articles 11 (1) (f) and 12, Convention on the Elimination of All Forms of Discrimination Against Women, 1979; Article 24, Convention on the Rights of the Child, 1989; and Article 25, Convention on the Rights of Persons with Disability, 2006.
117 Alicia Ely Yamini, Defining questions: Situating issues of power in the formulation of a right to health under international law, *Human Rights Quarterly* 18 (1996): 407.
118 Zahara Nampewo, Jennifer Heaven Mike, and Jonathan Wolff, Respecting, protecting and fulfilling the human right to health, *International Journal for Equity in Health* 21 (1) (2022): 1–2. https://doi.org/10.1186/s12939-022-01634-3.
119 V. R. Krishna Iyer, *A Judges Extra-Judicial Miscellany*, New Delhi: B R Publishing Corporation, 2011: 231; and United Nations, Economic and Social Council, *General Comment No. 14: The Right to the Highest Attainable Standard of Health*, Geneva: Committee on Economic, Social and Cultural Rights, 2000. www.refworld.org/docid/4538838d0.html.
120 Sheetal B. Shah, Illuminating the possible in the developing world: Guaranteeing the human right to health in India, *Vanderbilt Journal of Transnational Law* 32 (1999): 452.
121 Nishant Sirohi, Declaring the right to health a fundamental tight, *Expert-Speak Observer Research Foundation*, 14 July 2020. www.orfonline.org/expert-speak/declaring-the-right-to-health-a-fundamental-right/.
122 *Chandra Bhavan Boarding and Lodging v State of Mysore* (1969) 3 SCC 84.
123 Gautam Bhatia, Directive principles of state policy, in Sujit Chowdhary, Madhav Khosla, and Pratap Bhanu Mehta (eds.), *The Oxford Handbook of The Indian Constitution*, New Delhi: Oxford University Press, 2020: 650; n. 39 *Kesavananda Bharti*; *Minerva Mills v. Union of India* (1980) 3 SCC 635.
124 AIR 1984 SC 812.

125 AIR 1984 SC 812.
126 n. 7 *Duggal.*
127 n. 7 *Duggal.*
128 Anup Surendranath, Life and personal liberty, in Sujit Chowdhary, Madhav Khosla, and Pratap Bhanu Mehta (eds.), *The Oxford Handbook of The Indian Constitution*, New Delhi: Oxford University Press, 2020: 769.
129 Kajal Bhardwaj, and Veena Johri, Covid-19 vaccines in India: Judicial blind spots in upholding the right to health, *Socio-Legal Review* 18 (2) (2022): 119.
130 Shylashri Shankar, and Pratap Bhanu Mehta, Courts and socioeconomic rights in India, in Varun Gauri and Daniel M. Brinks (eds.), *Courting Social Justice: Judicial Enforcement of Social and Economic Rights in the Developing World*, New Delhi: Cambridge University Press, 2008: 147.
131 Aparna Chandra, A life of contradictions: Group inequality and socio-economic rights in the Indian Constitution, in Shreya Atrey and Sandra Freeman (eds.), *Exponential Inequalities*, Oxford: Oxford University Press, 2023: 318.
132 Dhingra Swati, and Maitressh Ghatak, The pandemic in data: How Covid-19 has devastated India's economy, *Scroll*, 9 May 2021. https://scroll.in/article/999275/the-pandemic-in-data-how-covid-19-has-devasted-indias-economy.
133 Vipin Bahadur Singh, The human costs of Covid-19 policy failures in India, *Nature Human Behaviour* 5 (2021): 810–11. https://doi.org/10.1038/s41562-021-01140-6.
134 Edouard Mathieu, Hannah Ritchie, and Lucas Rodés-Guirao et al., India: Coronavirus pandemic country profile—cases, *Our World in Data* (2024). https://ourworldindata.org/coronavirus/country/india.
135 Edouard Mathieu, Hannah Ritchie, and Lucas Rodés-Guirao et al., India: Coronavirus pandemic country profile—cases, *Our World in Data* (2024). https://ourworldindata.org/coronavirus/country/india.
136 Jacob Koshy, WHO estimates 4.7 million Covid-19-linked deaths in India, *The Hindu*, May 5, 2022. www.thehindu.com/sci-tech/health/who-estimates-47-million-covid-linked-deaths-in-india-10-times-official-count/article65385669.ece.
137 C. P. Chandrasekhar, The Indian economy before and after the pandemic, in Vikas Rawal, Jayati Ghosh, and C. P. Chandrasekhar (eds.), *When Government Fail—A Pandemic and Its Aftermath*, New Delhi: Tulika Books, 2021: 173.
138 The Wire Staff, Covid-19 blow: India's GDP shrinks by a record 23.9% in the first quarter of FY'21, *The Wire*, 31 August 2020. https://thewire.in/economy/india-gdp-record-shrinks-fy21-q1-covid-19-lockdown.
139 Radhicka Kapoor, The unequal effects of the Covid-19 crisis on the labour market, *The India Forum*, 15 July 2020. www.theindiaforum.in/article/unequal-effects-covid-19-crisis-labour-market.
140 Radhicka Kapoor, The Covid-19 pandemic pushed millions of Indians into poverty, *The Economist*, 12 January 2022. www.economist.com/graphic-detail/2022/01/12/the-covid-19-pandemic-pushed-millions-of-indians-into-poverty.

3 The Task Before Rebuilding

COVID-19 Second Wave in Jharkhand, Impact and Responses

Sushmita

The COVID-19 pandemic impacted multiple facets of the lives of people. As with most diseases, this too was felt differently by different sections of society. It became difficult to remain hopeful, in a crisis that unfolded variously across different sections of the society, and with things slipping out of government authorities' hands.

Even as I was still trying to understand the full effects of the first wave of COVID-19 in India, the second wave hit. I was initially engaged in rapid action studies and investigation of how the first wave impacted COVID-19 in the forest areas (Impact of COVID-19 Outbreak and Lock Down Measures on Tribal and Forest Dwellers, 2020)[1] (Sushmita 2020).[2] However, when the second wave of COVID-19 peaked, a sense of absolute chaos gripped us, as people reached out for support, amplification of messages on social media for oxygen support, emergency requests, availability of beds and more. My twitter inbox was flooded with many such requests, and it seemed like we were literally in the eye of the storm. I can still feel the effects of the time vicariously. This was also the time when vaccine was introduced and information about the vaccine was shrouded in propaganda and there was a lack of understanding[3] (Sushmita and Harsha 2023).

The first wave had already shown the effects of the pandemic on different sections of people, and my work on forests, climate and indigenous communities led me to understand and interact deeply with Adivasi and forest communities and document their specific problems (Sushmita 2020)[4] To that extent, literature suggested that Adivasis bear a "disproportionate burden" of communicable diseases in India, that includes diseases such as tuberculosis and malaria. Despite constituting only about 8 percent of the national population, they account for about 30 percent of all cases of malaria and 50 percent of mortality associated with it (MoTA 2014).[5]

Much before the pandemic broke out, an expert committee on Tribal Health, which had presented its report in 2014, said that it was particularly concerned that there was no "comprehensive plan for the development of tribal people, including health at the national level." The *Tribal Health Report—Bridging the Gap and a Roadmap for the Future* prepared by this Committee observed[6] the following:

DOI: 10.4324/9781003591641-5

"Unfortunately, the MoTA [Ministry of Tribal Affairs] does not lead the other departments in planning for various aspects of tribal development. Similarly, MoHFW [Ministry of Health and Family Welfare] or NHM [National Health Mission] did not actively consider for *[sic]* tribal health. Health of the most vulnerable was left out by both the ministries."

The report had noted that tribals in India faced triple burden of diseases, where there was rampant presence of malnutrition, disproportionately high incidence of communicable diseases like malaria and tuberculosis, and that there was a recent spurt in non-communicable diseases such as cancer, hypertension and diabetes. Additionally, due to less and disrupted access to clean water, good sanitation and soaps, barrier measures[7] (Bourdelais 2021) are already weak in Adivasi communities.

So, when the pandemic broke out, it percolated to these communities and societies and exposed the structural gaps and fissures in service delivery.

The various developments that took place around this time, need to be looked at as a whole—whether it was the return of the migrant workers,[8] an acute food crisis,[9] accessibility to medicines or vaccines, issues of livelihood generation or anything else. Like every disease and social problem, it is the access to welfare and relief measures and the rights of an individual at such times that make the outcome of such a crisis different. Such moments make one wonder if there was another way, a better way in which the crisis could've been prepared for or faced. Past experiences have shown that during such times, dissemination of correct information becomes a key to effective response and the control of the spread of the disease.[10] Such moments also have the potential to lay down key pointers for a new future, if attention is paid to the way in which things failed or didn't work.

As many Indian states were still reeling from the effects of the first wave of COVID-19, the pandemic having reached every state at different points, starting from the metropolitans and cosmopolitan hubs to the hinterlands, they were faced with the second wave of the pandemic (Sushmita and Harsha 2023).[11] There was a gap of at least four to five months before the onset of second wave was recognised. It will be well worth looking into the key factors that could've been done differently and if at all these would have made any difference. The first wave caused considerable damages in its wake and pushed the people already facing systemic violence and structural neglect to a further margin. For instance, many migrant workers were left with no option but to return to the cities despite facing the threat of disease and deaths, after having returned to their homes during the first wave.

The diversity in the geographies across the country and the people who inhabit them, combined with their structural location in the society, determined that different classes, castes, genders and states experienced it differently.

On May 11, 2021, the WHO classified the B.1.617 variant of the Coronavirus as a "variant of global concern"[12] (Nebehay and Farge 2021). People were still to recover from the harsh lockdown of the first wave, during which cities, small towns and rural areas were locked down. Workers from cities returned to their homes in rural and tribal areas, while factories and farm work boarded up. The first wave of COVID-19 spread considerable damage in its wake.

The second wave was marked by key features such as an impact on higher age, short supply of oxygen and ventilator, difficult ICU admissions and organ failures compared to the first wave[13] (Kapoor and Panda 2022).

As the pandemic moved from the cities to the interiors, the impacts on poorer and least developed states and marginalised communities began to show. Yet, the media failed to address a lot of gaps in reporting. An information asymmetry followed.

The disease spread rapidly in states like Jharkhand, mainly due to relaxation of quarantine norms after the first wave and a somewhat lackadaisical approach of the state authorities and the central government in trying to control the spread of the disease. In one conversation with an official from the health ministry in Jharkhand, who wished to remain anonymous, the person confided that the government was trying but the existing infrastructure was so dilapidated that every effort of the state government to control the disease failed.

Residing in the state at the time, and having an online presence, I received many requests to amplify the emergency requests during this period. This, and my access to local news and a closer view of the state-run hospitals, as well as private hospitals, and the fact that I was also engaged in an analysis of the second wave of COVID-19 on forest-based communities made it imperative for me to deeply investigate what was happening. It is also important to understand that states like Jharkhand have otherwise, during normal times, also faced the apathy of mainstream media[14] (Sushmita, upcoming). To that extent, this chapter tries to break the information asymmetry that many states, far from the centres of political drama and power, face. This is so important if we want to address a crisis like the COVID-19, as also outlined in the vision of this book.

Emerging literature has already shown the impact of the crisis cuts across other deeply embedded social issues, also relevant for India, such as migration, poverty and illness.[15] (Sharma et al. 2021). This chapter challenges any universal narrative of the experience of COVID-19 by shining a light on indigenous and forest-dwelling communities, who are remotely located and difficult to reach. For instance, migrant workers, who had returned home after the first wave, many of whom were Adivasis, had no option but to go back after a point, in the search for livelihoods[16] (Sushmita 2020). In that sense, the sense of loss, with which the book takes off, hasn't fully been comprehended.

As many as 50 percent or more from the Adivasi communities across India have been displaced from their traditional homes (Mahapatra 2018), with the 2011 Census recording nearly 32 percent decline in the number of villages with 100 percent Adivasi population between 2001 and 2011.

Bestowed with extensive forest cover and Adivasis constituting close to a third of the population of the state, Jharkhand has 40 percent of India's mineral resources. This has led to the forced displacement of people as time has passed and made Adivasi communities extremely vulnerable[17] (Sushmita 2020).

Jharkhand, an eastern state in India, has been bestowed with ubiquitous beauty and natural resources and was the witness to one of the first struggles for independence during the colonial rule in India, with Adivasi rebellions erupting in several parts of the state. The state, then part of undivided Bihar, because of the long history of struggles saw several legislations meant to ensure and protect the rights of the Adivasi and forest-dwelling communities here. However, the approach of governments, in post-independent India has been extractive and usually has only been eyed for its resources.

A constant plundering of resources, at the hands of vested corporate interests, and with the support of governments—both central and state—has given way to structural violence, in that the most marginalised people have been displaced, killed and deprived of their rights. Adivasis, who have been categorised as Scheduled Tribes in the Indian Constitution, comprise a significant population of the state accounting for close to 29 percent of the population. Despite its separation from Bihar, on the demands of a better state of being for Adivasis, resource diversion for development-related activities has remained abysmal, lacking in several aspects such as health.

3.1 Note on Methodology

This book chapter has been inspired by the testimonials of people collected during the COVID-19 second wave, as well as the daily tracking of media reports during the months between March and June, 2021. The people spoken to were representatives of indigenous community, civil society representatives, experts on forest and natural resource governance and others. Qualitative methodology has been made use of to understand and process the information collected because of a lack of precedent in the recent past. Even as I was conducting another impact assessment study, my location in Jharkhand, as explained earlier, made me curious about how the pandemic unfolded in the state. Another researcher Suraj Harsha and I started collecting and documenting various news reports, government directives, online news etc. Afterwards, I interviewed several civil society representatives and experts from Jharkhand and other areas.

3.2 Health in Jharkhand

Jharkhand is one of India's five poorest states[18] (indiastatjharkhand 2021). Jharkhand, over the 12 years between 2010 and 2012 spent less than the average amount spent on healthcare by states (RBI). It was also one of the states highlighted as having a "severe deficit of healthcare facilities" in the 15th Finance Commission Report in India.[19]

On average, one Primary Health Centre (PHC) in Jharkhand serves more than 90,000 people as against the norm of 20,000 in tribal areas *according* to the government's rural health statistics for 2018–2019.[20] This marks a 72 percent shortfall of PHCs in the state. Primary Health Centres are intended as the first points of contact between rural communities and the public health system. Community Health Centres (CHCs) are slightly larger intermediate health facilities that serve referrals from PHCs and are one step before tertiary district hospitals. A CHC is supposed to be equipped with laboratories, X-ray machines, round-the-clock delivery facilities along with medical specialists, technicians and nurses of the total sanctioned posts for specialists in CHCs and lab technicians in PHCs and CHCs, more than 90 percent and 58 percent, respectively, are lying vacant.[21]

In 2020, the Comptroller and Auditor General (CAG) had pulled up the government for not utilising close to 90 percent of its INR 100.31 crore funds allocated to it. The CAG also said that the district hospitals procured medicines from local vendors without quality testing in the absence of centralised purchased drugs.[22]

The data with the state health department shows that it has only 188 sanctioned CHCs, of which only 171 are functional. This is merely 68 percent of the total number required.

Though India's public health strategy requires that a health sub-centre should constantly engage with the villages and induce "behavioural change towards modern medicines," the engagement on the ground is far from regular and is often limited to immunisation for children.[23]

The situation of health and health workers in the state has remained abysmal, right from the higher pay rank officials guaranteed payment by the sixth pay commission to contractual labour staff such as the sanitation workers. This was reported in multiple instances, as doctors and staff went on strikes at different places just before the COVID-19 situation worsened. One can assume that there has been a general discontent among the health workers in the state, as also the extreme shortage of health facilities has been marred with corruption; however, COVID-19 in general also pushed this discontent to the fore. Sanitation workers went on an indefinite strike in Jamshedpur's MGM hospital to demand for regularisation of payments. Some had worked for as long as 18 years as contractual staff.[24]

3.3 Situation of the COVID-19 Second Wave in Jharkhand

After the first wave started to recede, and only by December 2020, the Jharkhand government allowed schools to function for the classes 10th and 12th for the upcoming board exams. By February, the schools were allowed to reopen for students above class 8. Colleges, coaching centres, cinema halls too were scheduled to reopen.

However, owing to the news of considerable spread and following in the footsteps of its neighbours—Bihar, Odisha and Chhattisgarh—the government was compelled to impose restrictions

End of February and in the early days of March, the vaccination drive had started for the age group of 60+ years across India and every state was allotted a certain number of vaccines, as notified by the central government, based on the number of people who were above 60 years in that particular state. Though the vaccination drive had started, not many people could be vaccinated in the state before the second wave. As things were reopening towards February end, it was becoming evident that the state hadn't foreseen one of the worst crises that was going to plague it in the coming months, claiming thousands of lives.[25]

On 3 March 2021, the government went on to remove time constraints for COVID vaccine slots thus enabling all private entities to run vaccination 24 hours a day.

The numbers of cases in Jharkhand were in single digits for a few weeks, and on 4 March 2021, Jharkhand reported zero deaths in the past 24 hours. Again on 11 March 2021, there were no COVID deaths reported. Vaccination was steadily becoming the norm and even Governor Draupadi Murmu publicly took the first dose of vaccine on 10 March 2021 (Kumar 2021).

While the cases were in single digits and zero deaths, in some of the government hospitals the doctors and sanitation workers were on a strike. On 12 March 2021, it was reported that some senior resident doctors along with junior resident doctors with arrears were on strike; they were then promised to be paid by the end of March. Ironically, on 13 March 2021, it was reported that all medical expenses of all ministers will be borne by the state government including their treatment outside the state in any private or super speciality hospital thus acknowledging the limited infrastructure in Jharkhand. A day later, on 14 March 2021, the sanitation staff of MGM hospital, were on strike with arrears of more than three months; no promises were made to the sanitation staff.

By mid-March, the cases started purging again and on 18 March 2021, the Chief Minister of Jharkhand, Hemant Soren, expressed concern over rising cases in Ranchi and Jamshedpur thus returning to enforcing stringent measures in the days to come. As per the directives, people found without masks were also to be penalised. Ninety fresh cases and zero covid deaths were also reported in the past 24 hours. With rising cases, the government, on 20 March 2021, declared one month of extra pay to the 'frontline medical workers' without defining who is included in this category, more importantly the sanitation workers. After 20 March 2021, there was a spree of health directives by both the state and the centre.

Come elections for states like West Bengal and Assam, few ministers from Jharkhand including Jharkhand's State Health Minister Banna Gupta visited both the states for canvassing/rallying. Additionally, not only were the vaccines oddly distributed within the states with unequal distribution and limited or selective awareness in certain tribal areas but also that the Cowin portal to book vaccine slots was slow for the month of March, as reported.

Many rural areas had almost no network and no access to medical facilities as well. Some of the Accredited Social Health Activists (ASHA) workers were visiting villages door to door to spread awareness about the vaccine but due to deep distrust around modern medicine systems, vaccination of the most marginalised tribal people became impossible.

By 22 April 2021, the fresh cases had risen to 5041 with 62 deaths. (*Hindustan Times* 2021) The status on the day showed that the total cases recorded in the state till then were 1,77,356 with total recoveries being 1,39,921. Active cases were 35,826 while the death toll had risen to 1,609.

COVID deaths recorded in the state jumped from 1,609 on 21 April 2021 to 4,085 on 11 May 2021. It means that Jharkhand saw 2,476 deaths in 20 days, which averages to over 100 fatalities a day despite lockdown measures being in place. In the same period, the neighbouring state Bihar, which has a population three times more than Jharkhand's, registered 1,473 COVID deaths (Srivastava 2021).

It is noticeable how things quickly deteriorated between 20 March 2021 and April first week. While several states reported that they are facing a vaccine shortage, Jharkhand too said that it had vaccine stocks left only to last 1–2 days.

Witnessing the second wave of COVID-19, India reported more than 1.2 lakh new infections, the highest single-day spike ever since the pandemic started. Amidst this rise, several states, including Maharashtra, Chhattisgarh, Odisha, Andhra Pradesh and Jharkhand, claimed that they were facing coronavirus vaccine shortage.[26]

By 17 April, 2021, the Jharkhand High Court said that the situation of COVID-19 was "pathetic" as the state headed towards an emergency. The court attributed this to non-availability of beds, oxygen-supported beds and lack of supply of medicines for home-isolated patients. Medicines intended to boost immunity, such as those of vitamin C, also were found to be unavailable, and specialised medicines, such as Remdesivir whose efficacy was warranted, also were reported to be out of stock.

While observing the critical situation of the pandemic in the state, the Jharkhand High Court Bench said,

> "there is a pathetic situation in the State of Jharkhand, due to non-availability of beds, oxygen supported beds and even the patients are not in a situation to live in isolation in the house since they are not made available with the required medicines due to non-supply of such medicines. While on the other hand, it has been informed to this Court that injections like Remdesivir and tablets like Favipiravir are being black-marketed."
>
> (Leaflet 2021)

Earlier, in a hearing on 13 April, 2021, the bench expressed its dissatisfaction observing the inadequate medical facilities in the Rajendra Institute of Medical Sciences (RIMS), Ranchi—a public health facility and a prominent government college. At the time it also noted the shortage of CT scan machines even as the COVID-19 cases were on a rise. It said that the "non-availability of CT scan machines in an institute like RIMS is a matter of serious concern" (Leaflet 2021).

While urban centres recorded the highest number of cases, all districts showed a significant rise in the number of cases and deaths since mid-April.

Further, there was also a marked difference in the access to services to scheduled and non-scheduled areas.[27]

3.4 COVID-19 and Adivasis

Despite a rising second wave, Adivasis and forest-dwelling community members hesitated to go to the hospitals for their treatment. Vasavi Kiro, who runs a small research centre on forest medicines, told me, "My husband also got Covid-19 but it was treated at home only. There have been multiple false reports around the areas where I work, which has also instilled a fear in the minds of those who are suffering from various ailments."

Kiro's statements highlighted several issues such as the lack of trust in the modern medicinal systems, a lack of reach of the specific health facilities and lack of access. She added, "One person who had Typhoid was kept in a Covid-19 ward, from there he was shifted to a private hospital and eventually to a military hospital where he died."

In many rural areas in Jharkhand, around the time of the second COVID-19 wave, that is, the months of March–June, diseases such as typhoid, malaria and jaundice were far too common. Since most of these have similar symptoms, this made life hard for those in these areas.

Every year, thousands of people in Jharkhand are infected by malaria.[28]

"People are drinking *kadhas*, taking steam and herbs and curing themselves at home as much as possible. There is a lack of awareness on basic precautionary steps to take. Kiro has regular visitors from villages such as Adki, Mandar, Jaratoli, Badam, Aara, horhat etc from the Namkum block.

The time between first and second waves wasn't utilised to build an understanding of the disease, Kiro felt. What are the symptoms, what is the reason for the second wave. We bore so much in 2020 but we didn't do anything."

"It has become clear that health is not the prime agenda of the government. And the fissures of the system that somehow existed, are more evident now. There are no beds, no Oxygen. Anyone who is recovering, is because of their own knowledge of local medicines, and not because of government efforts," Kiro told me at the time.

On 5 May 2021, the Jharkhand government issued a directive to test the people returning to these areas.

Many people opted for home medication and treatment during the time, without any evidence of effectiveness of such treatments. Sister Divya Maria, a nurse at the Caramel Hospital in the state's Mahuadandr district said, "A phenomenon that we observe is that most people opt for home medication and treatment in the first cycle of the disease. By the time they reach third cycle [of the disease] their situation has already become complicated." Maria adds that during the second phase, they had 10–12 COVID patients every day. These were the people who had decided to go for hospitalisation.

"A local seller told a social worker that every day he sold a minimum of three coffins during the past two months. And we have people who cremate as well as bury [their dead]. So, you can imagine, how many must have died," she added. Mahuadandr area has around 33,400 (45%) Christian, 15,500 Hindu (20.79%), 5076 (6.79%) Muslims while 78.7 percent of the total population (58,802) are Adivasis (categorised as ST as per government categorisation). Many deaths as well as sicknesses in these areas went unreported.

This also resonated with the fears that there was a massive undercounting of deaths during the time owing to factors. An investigation done by Reporters Collective, a collective of journalists working on politics and governance, found that 3,59,496 more people died than in a normal year in Rajasthan, Jharkhand and Andhra Pradesh where governments claimed that only 28,609 persons had died of COVID.

In other areas such as Palamau, with a large number of Adivasi population, and also a scheduled district, the problems were many. Since villages are devoid of any medical structures, people landed up in towns. In Hussainabad, Palamau, large-scale corruption was alleged by people on the conditions of anonymity. Regular medicines such as paracetamol were sold at INR 100–200. For a poor state, that is a lot of money. On a regular day, a strip of paracetamol costs INR 10. Testing reports were delayed and sometimes took a month or so. There were also cases of hoarding of oxygen cylinders reported from some of these areas. Moreover, because of an acute shortage of doctors, many with inadequate experience opened up medical camps. A local news portal reported issues of oxygen being injected through syringes.

Many areas lacked basic facilities such as ambulances.

Jharkhand Janadhikar Mahasabha, a coalition of various Jharkhand-based platforms highlighted that there was a vaccine scare in various villages. In the village Bada Lageya of Chaibasa, villagers documented a death after vaccination and in the absence of proper support after vaccination, people are now saying that they don't want the vaccines. In one such incident, people documented this.

Another issue that was common during the time was that many of these centres were using the rapid antigen tests, which has a higher rate of false negatives. While the guidelines stated the need for these to be verified by a gold standard RTPCR test, the lack of awareness around it made the process difficult.

The platform also highlighted the issue of vaccine shortage in the state due to the centre's callous approach to these states.

3.5 Impact on Livelihoods

Minor forest produce sale and collection is an important source of livelihood for Adivasis in Jharkhand. However, both the COVID-19 first and second waves coincided with the time of the forest produce collection. At this stage, some of the respondents said that the places where women's groups and Self-Help Groups were active could collect, process and sell the produce in the market place in normal scenarios. However, the sale had to be immediate as otherwise there was a danger of the forest produce getting wasted. Since the big traders weren't allowed to cross the district borders, especially from places such as West Bengal, a neighbouring state. They would especially trade in Kendu leaves, which is used to make country cigarettes. Owing to similar problems related to the sale and marketing of forest produce, activists in the region alleged that Adivasi and forest-dwelling communities lost 70–80 percent of their income.

The delay in collection of the forest produce was symptomatic of deeper issues. "This year [2021] people are so caught up with health issues and have been completely swept by that, that they may have not been able to focus on the systematic collection and sales of the forest produce. Nobody has brought it up with me yet," Kiro, who runs a research centre on forest medicines and is a Jharkhand-based activist, told me.

Even as people struggled with sale and distribution of minor forest produce, a government hand remained absent. "Any form of procurement of the minor forest produce by the government is not taking place. For instance, right now people are marketing the *beedi* patta (Tendu leaves), but this is happening through private sales" the Convenor of NREGA watch from Jharkhand's Latehar, James Herenj told me. Tendu leaves have a high revenue generation potential. The leaves are used to wrap tobacco and prepare *bidis* (a local cigarette). *As per* Ministry of Tribal Affairs' data, while the estimated production potential of Tendu leaves is INR 1,040 crores, its collection potential is INR 520 crores.

People bought the *beedi patta* for very cheap. '100 *pole* is being sold at INR 125, and one *pola* contains a bundle of 50 leaves,' James added. A lack of structure and coordination between the district administration and the panchayats—the village-level decision-making body was observed. For *Mahua*, another major forest produce, Herenj says that though the villagers sold it for INR 50 per kg, the same will be sold at INR 70 per kg by the traders and middlemen.

When the lockdown was lifted, rains had already started. This caused damage to Kendu leaves. "[R]ainwater is the deadly enemy of Kendu leaf because if the leaf gets the moisture, immediately it will be spoilt as it cannot be used for making beedi," said activist Sanjay Basu Mallick. Lack of storage spaces such as godowns led to further loss of produce. He said that there was no report of the produce being sold, marketed, unlike other years.

The government too didn't purchase the produce at a minimum support price and it was said that "one hand didn't know what the other hand was doing."

Despite the premonitions of this crisis, the Ministry of Environment and Climate Change—the nodal ministry that overlooks issues related to forest and climate change in India—issued an advisory on 30 April 2022 which restricted the forest dwellers' access to forests. Experts working on forests and natural resource governance that I spoke with during the time protested this.

"Considering that there is no evidence of transmission of COVID-19 from humans to wild animals in their natural environment, it seems more motivated from the intention of using this opportunity to restrict local people's entry and restrict their use and access rights. I think in these difficult times when people are struggling to save their lives, facing trauma of dead family members and relatives, having lost already limited sources of livelihood, no access even to minimal food in some cases," said Neema Pathak Broome, Programme Coordinator for the Conservation and Livelihoods Programme at Kalpavriksh and the South Asia Regional Coordinator for the ICCA Consortium South Asia, based in Pune, India.

Another expert, Giri Rao who heads the NGO Vasundhara, also argued that since people's access to forests [on which they depend for their livelihood and other needs] itself was restricted "they should have been compensated [for the loss]." He said that in 2020 there were meetings by the Ministry of Tribal Affairs (MOTA)—the nodal ministry—with the responsibility to ensure and look after the rights and well-being of tribals—on various issues including forest dwellers' and it issues several notifications, but in 2021 a similar thing hasn't happened. Instead, "MoTA is posting yoga fliers on its official handles," he had added.

The absence of government initiative may also be responsible for the spread of the disease to remote areas impacting the most vulnerable communities, Rao felt, thus pointing to crucial link between the livelihood and health crisis in these areas. Despite the fact that many tribal villages are remotely located, the second wave spread to even the remotest areas, Rao asked, "If weekly markets (*haats*) are already closed, how did Covid-19 spread to areas where people are already living remotely, unless someone from outside went into these villages? This could be the middlemen and traders who usually buy forest produce from the people." *Haats* are market places in village areas. Because of the distance between several villages, weekly markets are organised by the villagers for the sale and exchange of goods and produce. It is a common practice across several villages in remote areas.

In the absence of effective response to and relief measures for COVID-19, the situation worsened in these areas.

Our analysis showed that the absence of any credible government assessment and information on COVID impact on tribal communities has affected relief and livelihoods measures.

The collection season for tamarind, *Mahua*, and wild honey was already over while it was midway for Mahua seeds, Sal seeds, and Tendu seeds when this research was conducted. A lack of communication about how their produce will be procured is also something that has been a cause of concern for the women.

"Government instead of ensuring that scheduled tribes, other traditional local communities and pastoral communities are approached, their health monitored, treatment facilities, fodder for the livestock, veterinary services are ensured and that they are provided with daily wages including through forest produce that they have traditionally gathered and are provided with required rations, is restricting their access to even the natural resources which could come to their support in these times," Broome said. Further restrictions of access and use of forest resources was not only a violation of the forest rights but also a serious violation of human rights and constitutional right to life.

3.6 NREGA and Employment

To address the livelihood crisis in rural areas and provide social security, the Mahatma Gandhi National Rural Employment Guarantee Act (MGNREGA) was brought in 2005. Despite wage rates being low, many in the state depend on the scheme especially during lean seasons.

In June 2021, the Centre asked the States to split wage payments under the Act into separate categories for Scheduled Castes, Scheduled Tribes and others from the said financial year. This caused fears related to unnecessary complications in release of funds, exposing further uncertainties with the changes as highlighted by the NREGA Sangharsh Morcha, a body working on NREGA issues.

An analysis of wage payments in Jharkhand in April and May by a collaborative research centre of engineers, social workers and researchers, LibTech India found no differences in the time taken to pay SC/ST workers and others, indicating that there was no benefit for marginalised communities under the new system. Moreover, their analysis also highlighted that the Centre took 26 days to pay workers even after States generated fund transfer orders, as opposed to the stipulated seven-day period.

Despite the introduction of direct payment into bank accounts rather than at work sites, there are delays in wage payments and that they are never paid 15 days after the work is completed as required by the law; hence, the need wasn't to complicate the system further but simplify it and ensure reliable wage payments. The payment should be completed in two stages in 15 days after closing of the muster roll. However, it was found in Jharkhand that it took 26 days to release the fund.

During the second wave, when COVID significantly impacted the rural and scheduled areas, the focus and emphasis of the central government should have been to expedite the payment of wages, researchers pointed out. Not only should the payments have been made on time, but also experimenting without a justified rationale was difficult to comprehend.

"As our study demonstrates, not only has the experiment not yielded the desired results, but also that even in the beginning of the financial year when the programme should be flushed with funds, completion of stage two is taking three times more time than it should. The delays also stand in contravention of the Supreme Court order of May 18, 2018, in the Swaraj Abhiyan vs. Union of India case concerning drought. The Centre must calculate the delays and pay compensation to the workers for the full extent of delays (in both stages of the payment process)," Sakina Dorajiwala, a researcher with the study, said.

Wages of over 10 lakh workers in Jharkhand under the Mahatma Gandhi National Rural Employment Guarantee Act were not paid around the period, according to data on the scheme's website.

James Herenz, Convenor of the NREGA Watch, a civil society outfit monitoring lapses in MGNREGA projects across Jharkhand, said:

> "Wages of Jharkhand's NREGA workers are pending since 45 days as the central government has not released funds. At a time when workers should get additional income to support their families during the pandemic-induced lockdown, the government has failed to deliver even their hard earned wages. It is another failure of the Narendra Modi government amid the pandemic and shows it is insensitive to the plight of rural workers."

According to data accessed from the state rural development department, there are nearly 10.65 lakh labourers who have pending wages to the tune of Rs 10.48 crore.

3.7 Lack of Cooperation Between the Centre and the State

One would expect that such times of crisis may have warranted expedited support from the Centre. However, quite the opposite happened in Jharkhand, where the head of the state at the time was Hemant Soren from the Jharkhand Mukti Morcha party, an opposition party to the ruling Bharatiya Janata Party at the centre.

The then Chief Minister Hemant Soren said that neither did the central government leave it on the state to handle the situation nor did it handle it properly. The central government proved as an impediment in importing medicines.[29] Further, that all major decisions like oxygen supply, medical equipment and vaccines were taken by the central government. States like Maharashtra were well endowed to float global tenders for vaccines, while Jharkhand could not.

Despite being in need of 3.5–4 crore vaccines, the state had received only 40 lakhs by as late as May 23, when the said interview was published.

The state distrust deepened as people died after taking vaccines, and in the absence of adequate post-vaccine awareness and care, there was no counter to the disinformation floated around.

Frequent discrimination when people did try to access the government facilities or schemes also led to mistrust in the health systems and governance. People didn't feel safe.

3.8 Discussion

It appears that from the start, the gap and lack thereof in government's approach had started to show. The first wave caused a fatigue, leading governments and people to feel relaxed and even induced irresponsible and risky behaviours, for a pandemic that was far from over. Some of these behaviours included lack of social distancing, quarantines, opening up of public spaces, and some even entirely unnecessary events such as political rallies. Though there was a bombardment of propaganda, political messaging and information, people found it difficult to make sense of much of it. There was confusion and myths surrounding the dissemination of vaccines, and the existing mistrust of state machinery increased manifolds. It became clear that it was exceptionally hard to manage a pandemic of this nature, in a country where the central government was more concerned with self-aggrandization and political profiteering, through various measures. Not only this, the othering of states that didn't have the same political party in its charge, despite the exploitation and misappropriation of its resources time and again, laid bare the glaringly extractive nature of treatment meted to the state, making a mockery of the federal structure of the governance.

In the absence of state support, people resorted to medication on their own, corruption ensued and science was left at the mercy of politics and suffered consequences of bad governance. This was also evidenced in the ruling of the Jharkhand High Court.

All this goes on to show that the task before rebuilding is high and mighty.

The myths and suspicions of ringing plates and clapping were given leeway, while the government remained conspicuously missing from governance.

Our media analysis brings some of these issues to light. The analysis helps in showing the sudden rise of the COVID-19 cases, some of which may have been preventable, in the presence of right messaging and interest in reaching out to the most marginalised. We used this analysis to build on the other aspects of life of people and showed the disproportionate impact on indigenous and forest-dwelling communities, whose every aspect of life was impacted. Our analysis also simultaneously shows a weakened state that couldn't take care of its citizens. The treatment during COVID-19 in Jharkhand reconfirms the understanding of exploitation and extractive approach meted to the state and instils concerns that at moments of crisis, some states will be treated like the other and will be left to face the crisis on their own. State support remained absent not only from health but also from livelihoods of people.

It is clear that the COVID-19 second wave had a deadly spell in Jharkhand, more so for indigenous communities residing in the area. The lack of any documentation of the impact created the need for a proper documentation that can capture the plight of the people. The state government faced impediments posed by an already dilapidated health machinery and lack of access to health services to large populations, as also the apathy of the central government, as is indicated by several reports. The challenges in health were too specific to each group the COVID-19 impacted, as well as the geographical locations. Corruption at such a time was rife and made the situation of Adivasis and forest communities more precarious. They further faced the consequences of a lack of planning by the State government, even with the available resources. Some of government's own ministers fell extremely sick during the time and the condition quickly deteriorated within a span of weeks throwing the state into a crisis where it struggled for hospital beds and oxygen cylinders, apart from other things. The severe shortage of healthcare professionals impacted the rural and tribal population at many levels. While many didn't get access to vaccines and testing, there were also misinformation and lack of awareness. The full scale of the devastation needs to be further understood, but the crisis wasn't limited to health only. With their livelihoods closely linked to their access to forests, a gap was created where access to livelihood became extremely difficult.

Notes

1 Impact of COVID-19 outbreak and lockdown measures on Tribals and Forest Dwellers: Preliminary Assessment Report, 2020. http://fra.org.in/document/COVID-19%20Assessment%20Report.pdf.

2 Sushmita, Pandemic unleashes fresh hell for India's adivasis, *Dialogue Earth*, 16 December 2020. https://dialogue.earth/en/justice/pandemic-unleashes-fresh-hell-for-indias-adivasis/.

3 Sushmita, and Harsha, Suraj, Fending for themselves- adivasis, forest dwelling communities and the devastating second wave of Covid-19, *The Hindu Centre for Politics and Public Policy*, 24 March 2023. www.thehinducentre.com/the-arena/fending-for-themselves-adivasis-forest-dwelling-communities-and-the-devastating-second-wave-of-covid-19/article66640859.ece.

4 Sushmita, Pandemic unleashes fresh hell for India's adivasis, *Dialogue Earth*.

5 Ministry of Tribal Affairs, *Report of the High Level Committee on Socio-Economic, Health and Education Status of Tribal Communities of India*, Government of India, May 2014.

6 Ministry of Tribal Affairs, *Report of the High Level Committee on Socio-Economic, Health and Education Status of Tribal Communities of India*, Government of India, May 2014.

7 P. Bourdelais, The Covid-19 pandemic in historical perspective. *Historical Social Research, Supplement* 33 (2021): 302–15. https://doi.org/10.12759/hsr.suppl.33.2021.302-315.

8 N. R. Krishna, P. Sivakumar, S. Subramani, and S. I. Rajan, Covid-19, internal transitions and vulnerable citizens: Narratives of the migrant crisis in India during

the pandemic. *Review of Development and Change* 29 (1) (2014): 5–24. https://doi.org/10.1177/09722661241246837.
9 Nidhi Kaicker, Gupta Aashi, and Raghav Gaiha, Covid-19 pandemic and food security in India: Can authorities alleviate the disproportionate burden on the disadvantaged? Journal of Policy Modeling 44 (5) (2022): 963–80.
10 S. Sampath, A. Khedr, S. Qamar, A. Tekin, R. Singh, R. Green, and R. Kashyap, Pandemics throughout the history. *Cureus* 13 (9) (2021): e18136. https://doi.org/10.7759/cureus.18136. www.ncbi.nlm.nih.gov/pmc/articles/PMC8525686/.
11 Sushmita, and Suraj Harsha, Fending for themselves- adivasis, forest dwelling communities and the devastating second wave of Covid-19, *The Hindu Centre for Politics and Public Policy*, 24 March 2023.
12 S. Nebehay, and E. Farge, WHO classifies India variant being of global concern, *Reuters*, 10 May 2021. www.reuters.com/business/healthcare-pharmaceuticals/who-designates-india-variant-being-globalconcern-2021-05-10/.
13 M. Kapoor, and P. K. Panda, India's second Covid wave: How is it different from the first wave? (PS07.04 (578)) *International Journal of Infectious Diseases* 116 (Supplement) (2022): S50.
14 Sushmita, Analysis media coverage of an encounter killing of an Indigenous person in Jharkhand in June 2021, *TBD*.
15 J. R. Sharma, Anurag Sharma, and Anuj Kapilashrami, Covid-19 and the precarity of low-income migrant workers in Indian cities, *Society and Culture in South Asia* 7 (1) (2021): 48–62. https://doi.org/10.1177/2393861720975618.
16 Sushmita, Pandemic unleashes fresh hell for India's adivasis, *Dialogue Earth*.
17 Dev Nathan, Harishwar, Dayal, Resource curse and Jharkhand, *Economic and Political Weekly* 44 (51) (2009). www.epw.in/journal/2009/51/commentary/resource-curse-and-jharkhand.html.
18 IndiastatJahrkhand.com.
19 Prachi Salve, Despite increased spending, health outcomes remain poor in backward states, *Indiaspend*, 20 May 2022. www.indiaspend.com/health/despite-increased-spending-health-outcomes-remain-poor-in-backward-states-818516.
20 Rural Health Statistics, Government of India, Ministry of Health and Family Welfare, 2018–19. main.mohfw.gov.in/sites/default/files/Final RHS 2018-19_0.pdf.
21 Varsha Poddar, An old mistrust of the government keeps Jharkhand's adivasis away from Covid-19 vaccines, *The Caravan*, 30 May 2021, Why Adivasis mistrust Jharkhand's COVID-19 measures (caravanmagazine.in).
22 88 Percent funds not utilised: CAG slams Jharkhand on medical and health infrastructure, *Medical Dialogues*, 20 March 2022, medicaldialogues.in.
23 Varsha Poddar, An old mistrust of the government keeps Jharkhand's adivasis away from Covid-19 vaccines, *The Caravan*, 30 May 2021, Why Adivasis mistrust Jharkhand's COVID-19 measures (caravanmagazine.in).
24 Kumud Jenamani. Sanitation workers of MGM hospital go on strike, *Telegraph India*, 11 March 2021, Workers-protests—Sanitation workers of MGM hospital go on indefinite strike—*Telegraph India*.
25 Dhritiman Ray, 53% of all COVID-19 deaths in Jharkhand are senior citizens, *Times of India*, 9 June 2021. https://timesofindia.indiatimes.com/city/ranchi/53-of-all-covid-19-deaths-in-state-are-senior-citizens/articleshow/83350637.cms.
26 COVID vaccine: No shortage. 43 million doses in pipeline' says Harsh Vardhan, *Mint*, 8 April 2021, COVID vaccine: 'No shortage. 43 million doses in pipeline', says Harsh Vardhan | Mint (livemint.com).
27 Why Adivasis mistrust Jharkhand's COVID-19 measures (caravanmagazine.in).
28 Number of malaria cases across Jharkhand from 2014 to 2022, *Statista* India: number of malaria cases in Jharkhand 2021 | Statista.

29 Abhishek Angad, COVID-19 a national problem but states left to themselves, *Indian Express*, 23 May 2021, Hemant Soren Interview: COVID-19 a national problem, but states left to themselves (indianexpress.com).

COVID-19 Highlights: Jharkhand reports 5041 new COVID-19 cases, 62 deaths, *Hindustan Times*, April 2021.

Amitabh Srivastava, What's behind the rising COVID wave in Jharkhand, *India Today*, 12 May 2021 (indiatoday.in).

Sabrang India, Pathetic situation in the state, shortage of oxygen, beds and medicines: Jharkhand HC, *Leaflet*, 2021.

Part II

Migration, Indigeneity, and Cultural Impact

4 Navigating Medical Neglect and Care

COVID-19 Management and Adivasi Societies

Rashmi Kumari

4.1 Introduction

In the early summer of 2021, several Adivasi youths in the age category 18–45 of the population eligible for the COVID-19 vaccination were sceptical about getting vaccinated. As one of the youths, Barse Sunil had explained to me, 'The young men will not get vaccinated; in the village, boys are saying that they won't take the vaccine. They (social media messages) are saying only older men and women should get vaccinated. If young women and men get vaccinated, they won't become mothers and fathers'. Sunil is a 21-year-old Adivasi youth who volunteers with a local NGO to teach basic literacy to primary school children in Sukma, the southernmost district in Chhattisgarh. During the COVID-19 pandemic lockdown, Sunil also volunteered with the health department's efforts in 'contact-tracing'—a process of identifying individuals who had been in the proximity of a person diagnosed with COVID-19 in order to isolate, test, or treat them. Despite being in close to both the education and health department, Sunil was unsure of receiving the COVID-19 vaccination for himself.

Like Sunil, several youths received text and video messages on WhatsApp warning them of the consequences of vaccination, ranging from conspiracy theories to misinformation about the immediate and potential harms of vaccines. Although there were many rumours and myths about the COVID-19 infection and vaccinations floating in rural India, the fear and distrust among Adivasi communities of Sukma cannot be attributed to the fake news[1] created on social media alone. The fear of vaccination among the rural Adivasi population of South Chhattisgarh is rooted in historical encounters between the 'modern' health systems and the Adivasi communities.

In this chapter, I argue that COVID-19 was one among many crises that the Adivasi community has faced over the last century and that their suspicion towards taking vaccinations cannot be brushed under the popular perceptions of Adivasi being 'ignorant, superstitious, and innocent village folks'. Instead, Adivasi communities' reluctance should be understood along with the historical, political, and medical negligence of the state and the governing systems.

DOI: 10.4324/9781003591641-7

Further, the chapter shows that the Adivasi communities' distrust towards the state-administered healthcare services can be located in two larger practices: First, a firm belief in the efficacy of the local Indigenous healing systems and their ubiquitous presence. Second is the state medical system's historical absence and insensitivity towards the local population. While the former, I show, is a practice of care, the latter is experienced as physical and symbolic violence and what Bambra and others have called a 'syndemic pandemic'.[2] I show that the two aspects, care and violence, are interconnected with each other and exist in a continuum.

Additionally, I highlight these aspects of the existing parallel health systems in the Sukma district of South Chhattisgarh to demonstrate that the administrative management of the COVID-19 crisis only strengthened the divide between the two systems. The 'management' efforts resulted in pushing the Adivasi community away from the 'modern' medical services provided by the state and towards an increased belief in the local healing practices. I do this by sharing three vignettes around medical emergencies and the corresponding community responses I observed during the pandemic period in 2021. In these situations, I focus on the narratives offered by youth and community participants and their beliefs (and scepticism) in their Indigenous healing and therapeutic systems.

Exploring the long-standing interrelationships between care, neglect, and violence, my intention in this chapter is to underscore how the 'mismanagement of COVID-19 crisis'[3] is not a result of long-standing administrative neglect but an arrangement of multiple processes. I do not suppose that people were irrational in not believing in the virulence of the pandemic. Instead, I argue that containing the outbreak and the impact of a pandemic that remains mysterious at large was only a small part of the civic work undertaken by the government in a sea of neglected welfare work over the last century. The people's reluctance towards vaccination is not a sign of their irrationality or disbelief in modern medicine, vaccination, and the hospital system. It is rooted in their often 'cruel' and discriminatory encounters with the healthcare system; experiences have led them to doubt the health representatives' care efforts for the community.

I start the chapter with a brief discussion on the theoretical framework of the 'continuum of violence',[4] which I employ to demonstrate the tensions between medical neglect and existing health inequalities among Indigenous groups. This is followed by the section situating Sukma district, where I conducted ethnographic fieldwork from January to December 2021. The two sections contextualize Sukma in a more extensive political geography of the Indian State, which explains the Adivasi communities' perception of the district administration's management strategies for COVID-19. The third section weaves in the community perceptions of efforts made by the district administration in managing the second wave of the COVID-19 pandemic that hit the country during the summer months of 2021 and their Indigenous worldviews towards illness and cure. Offering three different kinds of health emergencies, this final part examines the interconnection between community's perceptions embedded in a traditional healing system in the region and long-standing medical neglect by the state administrations. By comparing the two medical systems, Indigenous and 'modern' biomedical health services, and the structures of marginalization entrenched in the latter, I argue that the COVID-19 pandemic is among many health emergencies that the communities in this area continue to face.

Moreover, as the introduction to this volume argues, the 'governance of the crisis' renders visible the medical marginality of the people of South Chhattisgarh at large, whose modes of care and experiences of neglect and violence emerge in the historical interrelations of state oppressions. I analyse the administrative response to the pandemic and the general attitude of the healthcare providers towards Adivasi communities' well-being within what Philip Burgois and Nancy Scheper-Hughes call a 'continuum of violence'.[5] In other words, I argue that in order to understand the impact of COVID-19 and its governance in the regions predominantly inhabited by Adivasi communities, it is crucial to recognize the interconnectedness of various visible and invisible forms of violence.

4.2 A Politics of Neglect in a Continuum of Violence

Nancy Scheper-Hughes and Phillipe Burgois proposed the concept of a 'continuum of violence' to explain that different forms of violence—symbolic,[6] structural violence,[7] spectacular forms of public violence[8]—are interconnected. Scheper-Hughes and Burgois write, 'Violence is . . . nonlinear, productive, destructive, and reproductive—as it gives birth to itself'.[9] In their explanation of the continuum, they compare it with the catchphrase 'like produces like' to contend that violence perpetuates itself, forming interconnected 'chains, spirals, and mirrors'[10] or what can be better understood as a continuous spectrum. Furthermore, violence extends beyond physical harm, encompassing assaults on the victim's sense of self, dignity, and worth. The social and cultural dimensions of violence imbue it with profound meaning and power. Therefore, a narrow focus on the physical aspects, such as force or pain infliction, overlooks its deeper implications. The authors in the edited collection *Violence in War and Peace* reflect on different forms within the continuum of violence and conclude that the concept of structural violence, encompassing poverty, hunger, and social exclusion, inevitably spills over into intimate and domestic spheres. Further, symbolic violence magnifies politically motivated violence such as torture, humiliation, stigma, shame, and in the act of being outcasted.[11]

The entanglement of the different forms of violence notably marks the lives of Indigenous communities and of the 'structurally vulnerable'.[12] The routinization of state violence in areas inhabited by Indigenous peoples also occurs in the form of neglect, which leaves people in prolonged precarity. Neglect is one of the most visible and recognized forms of violence, as it is stressed in many reports on the status of health, poverty, education, livelihood, and labour. However, it is essential to identify other forms of violence and their interdependency with neglect in the context of Central India, which has been the centre of a protracted civil conflict between the banned Communist Party of India (Maoist) and the Indian State. The insistent presence of violence transforms the lives of Indigenous peoples and their relationships with the state. Also, the recognition of violence is pertinent in understanding communities' interaction with the state around welfare, including the management of pandemics like COVID-19.

The present-day Sukma is an exemplar of this continuum where violence manifests in structural, physical, symbolic, and slow forms whose impact is experienced every day by the communities. It is this every day state violence, and especially in the forms of neglect, that I focus on in this chapter. The everyday state violence is further characterized by the 'social production of indifference'[13] or a 'normalized violence'[14] as it manifests as a routine occurrence in the lives of marginalized communities. This routinization of state violence against the rural poor occurs in the form of a 'normal absence of state provisions'.[15] This state neglect that Adivasis face is in the form of malarial deaths, long suffering from tuberculosis, malnutrition and starvation, and lack of essential health services.

In addition to the structural violence that reveals itself visibly in health inequalities, Adivasi communities experience symbolic violence. Symbolic violence occurs through the misrecognition of communities that are subjugated.[16] The trace of colonial othering of the present-day Adivasi communities takes place when colonial violence is replaced by everyday bureaucratic violence[17] in the forms of continued marking of the communities and in classifying the entire area as 'backward'. The misrecognition of violence occurs among the Adivasi communities when there is an 'internalization of innate failure'[18] among the people who, for centuries, have been politically othered.

I analyse the COVID-19 management efforts by the state and district administration in the backdrop of the aforementioned competing forms of marginalization. The communities' perception of the COVID-19 pandemic and its management efforts is an important insight towards the existing poorer health outcomes among Indigenous people across the world. Studies have shown, both globally and locally in India, a low life expectancy at birth, high mortality among infants, and increasing levels of malnutrition and stunting of Indigenous children.[19] Additionally, there is a high prevalence of neglected tropical diseases such as malaria, tuberculosis, sickle-cell anaemia, and dengue, among others.[20] These poorer health indicators add to the higher rate of mortality, morbidity, and malnutrition which worsened during the COVID-19 pandemic.

Examining the implications of the COVID-19 pandemic and health inequalities, Bambra and others argue that the most disadvantaged communities' experiences of the pandemic must be looked at as a syndemic pandemic.[21] The concept of the syndemic pandemic was developed by Merrill Singer, who analysed the relationship between risk factors and comorbidities of the HIV/AIDS pandemic in the 1990s USA. Utilising the concept of a syndemic pandemic, Bambra and others argue that in 'the most disadvantaged communities, COVID-19 is experienced as a syndemic—a co-occurring, synergistic pandemic that interacts with and exacerbates their existing NCDs and social conditions'.[22] The experiences of Adivasi communities of Central India, where the infection rates were perceived as not so high,[23] and the infection was also described to be 'milder' in comparison to the other parts of the country, the impact of COVID-19 is beyond virus-related infections. It must be looked at in the overall relationship between the pandemic, the social determinants of health inequalities, and the economic crisis caused by the sudden nationwide closures.[24] I argue that Adivasi communities' experiences of the pandemic must be analysed within this nexus of existing health inequality, persisting poor governance and infrastructure in the socio-economic well-being of the communities, and a crisis on subsistence livelihood practices imposed by the sudden lockdown. Further, in a context of conflict and militarization, existing socio-economic and health precarities are intensified.

4.3 A History of Neglect in the Adivasi-Dominant Areas of South Chhattisgarh

Sukma, the southernmost district of Chhattisgarh, was part of the formerly princely state of Bastar. Bastar, a single district in Madhya Pradesh, was divided into three districts, Kanker, Bastar, and Dantewada, in 1998. With the carving out of Chhattisgarh state from Madhya Pradesh in 2001, Bastar province was further subdivided into present-day seven districts. Sukma was formed in 2012 by partitioning the Dantewada district into two. While the entire Bastar province, and especially Sukma, has been famous for the protracted civil conflict between the banned Communist Party of India (Maoist) and the Indian State, the parent Chhattisgarh state, with the most abundant mineral reserves in the country, consistently remains to be labelled as a 'backward' region. Predominantly inhabited by Adivasis (83%) and with a forest cover of 65%, the district Sukma is also considered as one of the districts with the lowest literacy rates (35%) in India.

Nandini Sundar explains that while there was an 'increase in state-expenditure on schools, roads, and hospitals' in the larger Bastar region during the post-independence period, extraction of mines and timber from this region had also increased.[25] Treating the region solely for extraction has continued since colonial times. A recent influx of multinational corporations interested in the appropriation of Indigenous land and forests for commercial use resulted in a spate of 'developmental' projects.[26] The impact of this relationship between the state and the international agencies produced a 'simultaneous and contrary development',[27] leading to 'disempowerment and fragmentation alongside empowerment, cohesion, and politicization'.[28]

Further, the region, along with other Adivasi areas of peninsular India, is identified as 'development sites suited for building multipurpose river projects such as mines, thermal power, and paper factory that cause displacement of Indigenous people from their land and resources. Indigenous communities' experience of the state, since colonial times up until now, has been one of police brutality and violence'.[29] Though the communities have struggled against state oppression over the centuries, their recent discontent towards the state transpired under the leadership of the armed guerrillas of the Communist Party of India (CPI (M)), also known as Naxals.[30]

Violence in Chhattisgarh has a more extensive history that I do not have the space to discuss here. However, post-2000, the area faced a civil uprising against the people's government of CPI(M) and heavy militarization of the entire Indigenous areas of Central and Eastern India. Sundar quotes human rights activists to draw connections between the liberalization of India's mining policies[31] and state-supported violence. The local Adivasis of Chhattisgarh state faced a regime of terror[32] that ensued when the armed vigilante group under the banner Salwa Judum (literally meaning 'purification hunt' in Gondi) burnt houses and forced people from their homes either into the 'relief camps' which were heavily surveilled by the vigilante or into the forests under the protection of the Naxals, disrupting their centuries-old traditional lifeways.[33]

In the last two decades, the Bastar area, which an earlier prime minister called the 'gravest threat to the internal security of India',[34] saw intense militarization through Central Reserve Police Force (CRPF) camps, colloquially called police camps. More camps are being added every year. There are over 45 Forward Operating Bases in the province with an area of ten thousand square miles.[35] Although heavily armed, these camps have mottos such as 'peacekeepers of the nations', 'a step towards non-violence', and 'serving you, every step of the way'.[36] An intense militarization with a message of peacekeeping confounds state oppression in the language of care.

Over these years, along with the police presence, the district has also seen an increase in health centres and healthcare workers. The district's website boasts one district hospital, three community health centres, and 15 primary and 95 subhealth centres. Apart from the state's formal initiative in healthcare services, the CRPF bases also conduct health and well-being camps. Nevertheless, the official health workers and NGO volunteers during my fieldwork described the fund crunch the district hospital faced at the time. Moreover, the corruption within and between departments[37] and their limited reach in the villages occupied/inhabited by the People's Liberation Guerrilla Army of the CPI (Maoist) remains a challenge for a functional healthcare system.

4.4 Experiences of Health Emergencies as a Medical Neglect Within the Continuum

In addition to structural and politico-economic factors, Adivasi communities in Sukma face two distinct challenges. One, there has been poor access to the 'beneficial' policies and projects until recently, and two, the policies in place are structurally discriminating with limited civic infrastructure, lack of proper funds, corruption in various departments, and finally, discriminatory and casteist attitude of predominantly non-Adivasi service providers towards Adivasi patients.[38] Speaking of welfare policies and neoliberal projects on health, there have been targeted state-sponsored programs in maternal health and the prevention of malaria, tuberculosis, and sickle-cell anaemia. In response, civil society organizations have recently started services for trauma and mental health issues of children affected by conflict. Without a comprehensive state infrastructure in rural Central India, independent doctors trained in community health and NGOs, including the Médecins Sans Frontier (MSF), have provided preventive and curative healthcare in Bastar and other rural parts of India.

However, with the growing intensity of the armed conflict between the Maoists and the Indian State in the early 2000s, the district healthcare workers have hesitated to work in the rural areas, and the work of the NGOs and independent doctors has come under strict scrutiny and surveillance. Under a series of surveillance and control strategies, the Indian State arrested the famous paediatrician and human rights activist Dr Binayak Sen[39] and directed the MSF practitioners to restrict their services to paramilitary camps and areas supervised under them.[40] It left a large part of South Bastar that is often called 'Maoist strongholds' in journalistic circles outside of medical access. With a halt in the work of many rural health clinics in the area, upon his bail two years later, Dr Sen called the neglect in health care a structural violence. Sen explains this, 'by structural violence, I refer to the fact that half our children and our adults in this country suffer from malnutrition. Malnutrition casts a dark shadow over other diseases like malaria and tuberculosis. For example, a study by the National Nutrition Monitoring Bureau says that more than 60 per cent of Scheduled Tribes have a body mass index (BMI) of less than 18.5. According to the World Health Organisation, if more than 40 per cent of the population of a community has a BMI of less than 18.5, the community can be considered to be in a condition of famine. A third of our live births have low birth weights. This is what I mean when I talk of structural violence'.[41]

In the decade between 2006 and 2017, although the state seized most of these areas under its control using militarization strategies, healthcare access to rural communities remains in appalling condition. The Lancet–Lowitja Report on *Indigenous and tribal peoples' health* reported that, with a higher prevalence of poverty among Indigenous groups, India exhibits an Indigenous life expectancy at birth lower than 65 years, whereas there is a persistently high rate of infant deaths (greater than 50 per 1,000).[42] It is in this scenario that the arrival of COVID-19 wreaked havoc over the area and forced a significant percentage of the Indigenous population towards loss of income and subsequent food insecurity.[43]

4.5 The Second Wave of COVID-19 Pandemic and the Adivasi World

It was around the end of March 2021 that the news of the second wave had started circulating. The eighth standard student-participants of my research, whom I accompanied in the *Mohalla* (neighbourhood) schools, started discussing that there would be another lockdown. The already scarce numbers of teachers in these alternative arrangements of *Mohalla* schools had started dwindling. By the middle of April, a partial lockdown was in place, which was extended to full lockdown by the end of the month. Although cases were not that high in early summer, the entire Bastar province of Chhattisgarh state went into full lockdown for the three months of May, June, and July. This was aided by the news of the second wave—the Delta wave—of the pandemic in the neighbouring state of Andhra Pradesh and its subsequent lockdown that forced thousands of Adivasi migrant workers to return home to Chhattisgarh. Sukma district, situated on the borders of Andhra Pradesh, Telangana, and Odisha, was particularly affected by the pandemic policies in these states.

Many young Adivasis travel to the nearest states for different migratory work. The lockdown policies not only forced these people to return home but also created added pressure on the district administration to control the migrating populace while also managing infection rates. Returning migrant workers also posed an additional challenge to the district administration as they could bring infection into the pockets that might otherwise be untouched by the virus. There were multiple checkpoints starting from borders at state, district, and even village levels. While the administration created a team of civil and health volunteers to maintain isolation protocols and contact tracing, village governments were instructed to create their own quarantine mechanisms. Many villages were reported to have created barriers of wood logs barring outside vehicles from entering. Each village council had appointed volunteers of both *panchayat* (governance) members, auxiliary nurse-midwives (ANMs) locally referred to as *mitanin*, and community (Adivasi) health workers to monitor every new person coming into the villages and grant entries only if they did not display COVID-related symptoms.

However, in a region where there are more paramilitary soldiers than civilians on the road, the rules and guardsmen, regardless of their social locations, are perceived (and experienced) as oppression rather than a pandemic management strategy. Moreover, for the villagers, COVID-19 was an illness that was spreading in the cities and not in villages. They believed that the villages were not as polluted as the cities and the disease would not spread there as it did in urban spaces. During one of the lockdown days, in a conversation, Podiyam Sakalu says that

> it is the comfort of the cities, in their air conditioning is where this Corona is spreading. Here in the village, we live in open, and not in enclosed walls. There are trees and fresh air. Villagers are hardworking people and that gives us strength to fight this disease. This is anyway like a flu, a cold, and some cough. We villagers are not weak like the city folks.

This widespread belief that the illness caused by COVID-19 was an 'outside' disease and that the villagers had immunity to fight common cold and flu-like symptoms also made them defy the lockdown rules. The fear of the police made the villagers defy the restrictions and the isolation period of two weeks for the ones found positive at various borders. They were particularly afraid of being held at isolation camps, comparing it with random picking by police and being in custody that have become routinized protocols of peacekeeping. Hence, the barriers did not stop them from crossing villages and even state borders through the connected jungle routes to which the villagers were well accustomed. This aided the spread of the infection and, in turn, made the restrictions more stringent.

This period also coincided with the province's efforts in its vaccination drive. Having received vaccines before other states, the state government flaunted its 'full vaccination' drive in the area that was already infamous for lagging in health services.[44] The staff at the Sukma District hospital (the only hospital in the district with three health centres across three blocks) and at the collectorate were actively vaccinating the villagers. The only medical van, which also doubled as a makeshift ambulance, transported vaccines and health workers across different villages each day. The initial phase of vaccination, after prioritizing the health workers, focused on the 'vulnerable population' above the age of 45. However, the staff in Sukma who went to the 'Maoist-stronghold' villages administered the vaccines to everyone above 18 years who came forward. This was in response to their fear of restrictions on accessing the villages multiple times due to the ongoing conflict. The health workers I spoke to during my fieldwork confided in me that this was the first time that anyone from the health department had ever visited some of these locations in over a decade. 'The old villagers understand the vaccine as giving them "*takat*" (strength injection). Some of the old men came forward asking for "*takat*" injections. However, there were villages from where everyone fled from their houses and hid in the forest the moment they heard the sound of the approaching medical van'.

The staff at the NGO, which I temporarily called home during the initial phase of the pandemic in 2021, volunteered to do contact tracing and update the database of infected people every day. The founder of the NGO, in an informal conversation, mentioned to me that the district was struggling to secure pulse oxygen monitors and personal protective equipment for all medical staff. Further, the district had no testing centre/laboratory or equipment. Every sample that was being collected was sent either to Jagdalpur, a town that is about 100 km from Sukma, for a rapid antigen test, which was not often accurate, or to the labs in the state capital in Raipur, about 500 km from Sukma, for the more reliable RTPCR test. A person with an infection took between a week to ten days to obtain a confirmed test result and necessary medication afterwards. The delay in the process and lack of transparency discouraged the villagers from testing even if they developed full symptoms.

The information around infection and vaccination triggered a deluge of floating folklore in villages and towns in this part of the country, which varied in its contents from Adivasi to non-Adivasi residents. The merit of the vaccination and that of the pharmaceutical company manufacturing and distributing the vaccination became a topic of everyday discussions. While the predominantly non-Adivasi staff at the NGO discussed the cases of vaccine failure resulting in unexpected health emergencies (and deaths in rare cases) in other parts of India, the Adivasi communities discussed fertility issues associated with vaccines. Referring to the medical neglect and poor health management that have resulted in the deaths of women in Chhattisgarh, this fear was not unsubstantiated, especially for a community that has witnessed a 'dubious history of sterilization'. Reports of women's deaths in mass sterilization drives in 2016 and subsequent years and similar directed medical interventions that were opaque to the community members triggered a concern. Sunil and other youths' response towards COVID-19 vaccination comes in the wake of these uninformed medical interventions that have harmed the community in more ways than gaining their trust. Moreover, there have been many instances of Adivasi communities being mistreated in the district hospital. In the next section, I present three health emergencies and associated community practices to demonstrate the unequal relationship between the 'modern' medical system and Adivasi communities.

4.6 Between Indigenous and 'Modern' Biomedical Systems

I helped Sabita get medical help from the district hospital several times during my fieldwork. During one such visit, when Sabita was admitted for deficient haemoglobin levels, a condition of sickle cell anaemia, she was visited by her uncle, who is also a *wadde*, an Adivasi healer. Her uncle wanted to ensure that he could also perform a healing ceremony while she was in the hospital. However, the hospital administration refused to allow the healer to perform such ceremonies. The administration insisted that 'the family was free to take Sabita home if they believed they could provide her with better care using the traditional healing methods'. Sabita's healer uncle returned to his village feeling insulted. In highlighting this incident, I intend not to compare the two disparate medical practices but rather to highlight the mistreatment and disrespect the community members experience in 'modern' medical establishments.

The above-described disrespect and othering of the Indigenous knowledge system and its experts are embedded in the modern and casteist medical system often dominated by the communities with caste and class privileges. Virginius Xaxa writes that the 'territorial privileges and rights are freely recognised in respect of the dominant communities in India, the same is denied to the tribal communities. In the process they are progressively getting dispossessed of their control over land, forest, water, minerals and other resources in their own territory and are increasingly subjected to inhuman misery, injustice and exploitation'.[45] Adivasi communities' value and knowledge systems are constantly evaluated using the deficit approach.[46] According to the deficit approach, while the Adivasi culture is described as 'backward', superstitious', and often merely 'exotic', the 'perceived underachievement among Adivasi youth is often explained as the failures of the entire community'.[47] The marginalization of Indigenous knowledge of treatment has also occurred in the anthropological and historical medical literature. Despite India being described as a space for 'thriving medical pluralism' *[iv]*, which includes medical systems such as Ayurvedic, Siddha, and Yunani traditions, Adivasi healing and treatment practices have been portrayed as 'little traditions'.[48] The therapeutic forms, often described as outside the biomedical forms, practiced in Adivasi-dominated areas are clubbed with religion and discussed as 'rituals and spiritual forms of treatment'.[49] Further, Helen Lambert shows that there are significant hierarchies among the therapeutic practices within the prevalent medical pluralism in India and that 'non-codified and subaltern therapeutics' that are often referred to as 'cultural aspects', 'folk tradition', 'healing', 'religion', 'ritual', or 'superstition' are left outside the domain of a medical knowledge system.[50]

Nevertheless, despite the peripheralization of the Adivasi therapeutic systems and centring of biomedicine, there have been times when the medical infrastructure's delayed action on repeated visits and appeals by the community members has resulted in loss of lives. In one such instance, a college youth, Mandavi Daso, learned that his entire village, situated at a distance of 20 km from the block health centre, was suffering from fluoride poisoning. Daso, an undergraduate student of sociology and geography and one of the youth participants in my research, shared the story of his village with me. For the last few years, there had been unexplained deaths in his village. Most of the deceased showed similar symptoms of 'weakness, fever, and swollen limbs'. Daso narrated to me that when several members of the village head's family died of this unknown disease, a few others visited the physical health centre in the block. The doctors paid no particular attention to the situation and returned the patients with generic medicines such as painkillers and vitamins. Finding no help from the hospital, a few members fled the village while others approached an Adivasi healer, a *wadde*. The *wadde* explained the situation as the wrath of an angry deity left unappeased during the long conflict years and that it would take a long time to propitiate the deity. Even after initiating the appeasement process, the deaths and illnesses continued. Having lost all hope, the villagers held a protest rally at the hospital, leading to the formation of a health committee team. It took almost three years since the first death for the team to visit the hamlet and for them to test the water for fluoride poisoning. I narrate the story of Daso's extended family navigating this severe health hazard with both the modern medical system and traditional healing system to highlight that this is one of many villages across Central India where the environmental destructions have worsened the already precarious health situation in the area.

What Sabita's family experienced is a form of epistemic violence, the occurrence of which is normalized to the extent that even the Indigenous healers and medicine people have neither internalized it nor entirely refused to engage with the biomedical system. Later, when Sabita's mother-in-law was hospitalized due to a third-degree burn accident, her healer relative refused to visit her in the hospital. The older woman insisted on being discharged from the hospital as she wished to be among her family and passed away soon after her discharge from the hospital. It is not the 'cultural barrier'[51] but the disrespect and epistemic othering that stops many Adivasi people from accessing the biomedical system.

Daso's experience is of slow violence—another aspect within the continuum. According to Rob Nixon, slow violence, as opposed to being hyper-visible, occurs gradually. As delayed destruction is scattered across time, slow violence is felt in the forms of environmental degradations, unchecked mining projects, and displacements of communities from their lands to enable corporate exploitations of natural resources.[52] The impacts of environmental degradation are particularly experienced by community members who live with the mining dust and with the altered chemical composition of the river water and underground water because of long years of mining. Communities living around coal mines in Central India are at an increased risk of acute respiratory infection (ARI), tuberculosis, and skin-related ailments.[53] Moreover, the mining dust also impacts agricultural and local forest produce, resulting in restricted food options. There have been many news reports and studies on the poisoning of groundwater or finding excessive levels of fluoride in groundwater. While the existing rock formations contribute to the presence of arsenic fluoride[54] in groundwater, excessive mining activities have contributed to the contamination of water above the ground. These contaminations have serious health implications. Any resistance to these development projects like mining results in the militarization of the area with consequences such as imprisonment, assault on the young, and labelling any resistance as a rebellion.[55] The COVID-19 pandemic and its management by the administration is part of a larger and interwoven politics of care and violence that marks the life of Adivasi communities. I demonstrate this nexus between care and violence and a larger dependence on the community for the former in the third health-related vignette from the field. I show that in the absence of enough state infrastructure, communities depend on each other for the necessary care.

4.7 Interrelations of Care and Violence

The blue tarpaulin huts starkly contrasted with the brown hills and green forests in the incessant monsoon rain. One behind the other, lining the two sides of a cleared mud track of the proposed site for the road, the tarpaulin huts were the face of the community resistance. Every old and young person there had come to resist the construction of the road aided by (and for) the militarization, as they participated in the sit-in rally every morning and chant slogans—take back the police camp! In the middle was a bigger hut that joins two tarpaulins—the organizers' hut. Walking up to the hut, I saw several youths huddled around a wooden cot. A young woman, Gangi, was lying on the cot—looking exhausted, with beads of sweat on her forehead and a thermometer sticking in her mouth. Oonga, another youth sitting by her side, had a malaria kit in his hand and was waiting for the test kit to show the result. 'You will be fine by tomorrow', he said to her before turning to me to explain how the kit works.

Administering tests and medication is taken as a collective responsibility and is arranged along with other temporary domestic chores among the youth protestors. Care as a collective responsibility could also be observed in everyday tasks of protesting and surviving the violence. While young women walk to the river in a group for their daily ablutions, young men go together to gather food grains from other villagers. Children take up the work of cleaning, serving, collecting firewood, collecting medicinal plants, fetching potable water, and leading the evening communal dances.

Similar to violence, care also exist in a continuum. One continually responds to the other. Exploring care and abandonment in self-medication by using antidepressants, among other medications, in the everyday intimate scenes in Chile, Clara Han offers the concept of affective configuration. The affective configurations, for her, are the familial arrangements and 'domestic decision-making on the care and neglect of family members'.[56] For Han, concerns of care 'were not posed in relation to a fixed ideal of the normative family or it is opposite the non-normative kinship relations . . . care was implicated in the norms of everyday lives, in the works of everyday domestic relations, the stakes in concealing need, the delicate struggles over intimate relationships in which body was staked, or the small neglects and denials that also made everyday lives'.[57]

'We have all the medical supplies here with us for malaria, flu, common cold and cough, and iron supplements for sickle cell anaemia', Oonga tells me. Oonga, as an active Adivasi youth in his community, received one day of training in administering simple medical tests. The training was conducted at a community health centre where village health workers, auxiliary nurse midwives (ANMs), and willing volunteers were trained in a few aspects of community healthcare. They were provided malaria kits, vitamins, antibiotics, paracetamol, millet protein, and mineral supplements. Usually, this supply is stored with the local ANMs, who are often from the Adivasi communities. However, here in this village, which has become a literal site of the frontier between the state paramilitary troops on one side and protestors on the other, divided by concertina wires, every household and protest hut inhabitant has their medical supplies.

I also remember seeing a transparent polythene (plastic) bag full of different tablet strips hanging on a bamboo pole of the thatched roof house of my middle-aged host. When asked about the bag, she smiled and told me that the supply of medicines was for the youth protestors. Back in the tarpaulin tent, the lines on Gangi's test kit showed that she was still infected with malaria and that she had to fight back the fever, the chills, and body-breaking aches for another day before the next test would be administered. Like Han's ethnography in Chile, the state of Central India has displaced the responsibility of care. The use of tests and self-medications in Sukma, like the use of antidepressants among families in La Pincoya, Chile, exist within the 'modes of care, neglect, and violence emerging from the interrelations and disjuncture of state programs, and intimate relations'.[58] Here, neglect is not as prevalent in the community's relations as it is in the relationship that the state shares with Adivasis. In addition, the Adivasi communities in Sukma also practice a parallel Indigenous system of healing, which is diffused with the modern biomedical system.

Han traces the enmeshed relationship of care with economic pressures that constrain and limit the experiences of care. In her book, she presents examples such as desires to care for kin with mental illness are met with limited economic resources or the normalization of self-medication of aches and pains from unstable work conditions and indebtedness. Han writes that care is diffuse, not definable in a simple way, and attending to it 'is similar to attending to violence in which contests around the question of what can be named as violence is a sign of something important at stake'.[59] For Han, attending to care as a problem in everyday life rather than as a category with defined borders has implications for the moral fabric of self-making. It is in these implications that limits of care are experienced. For me, violence and care are intimately tied to the very survival of the community, where survival itself is layered within institutions. The institutions described in the previous section contribute to the cycles of violence. There are two layers of interlinked work of care and violence, which I locate in Adivasi communities of the present-day Sukma. First, I have attempted to map linkages between the violence inflicted by human intervention in nature and the everyday forms of care that exist and emerge in relationalities against this kind of violence. Two, the linkages between violence and care found in the Indigenous cosmology and how it informs and influences people's attitude towards the pandemic situation that COVID-19 created. I will follow this second link in the next section.

4.8 Illness, Ill-Fate, and the Adivasi Cosmology

During the paddy cultivation season, I attended an appeasement ceremony performed by the Durwa community. A partial lockdown was in place due to the second wave of the COVID-19 pandemic. Villagers were discouraged from gathering in large groups, meaning no village festivals, weddings, or ceremonies could occur. However, this was also the season when weddings, appeasement of village deities, and other similar festivals took place. As I explained in the above section, villagers, believing that COVID-19 was a disease brought into the villages by outsiders, continued defying some of the COVID-19 protocols. On this Tuesday afternoon, when I arrived at the appeasement ceremony, I gathered that there was an unease in the group. The village elders explained to me the importance of the ceremony.

> It is performed every three years to appease the goddess of smallpox and chickenpox. We have been performing it since our ancestorial time. If we do not perform it this year, we will have to wait for another three years to perform this again. The deity will get angry, and she might harm us with causing fever, measles, and other ailments.

Writing about the Indigenous belief systems on illness and death among Adivasi communities, Nandini Sundar writes, 'In Bastar cosmology, nothing happens of itself—everything is caused by deliberate action. Things proceed smoothly because the earth and mother goddesses are satisfied with the sacrifices that humans have made. Unexpected or unnatural disasters are caused either by deities who are unappeased or by the malevolent and random action of evil spirits or unsatisfied ghosts. There is no sharp distinction between good and evil forces—the same deities who ensure prosperity can also cause harm if angered; similarly, the same people who cure can also cast spells through the power of their Devi. Illnesses are usually diagnosed by a *siraha* (shaman or medium) or a *wadde* or *gunia* (herbal healer)'.[60]

In the performance of care, the village elders defied the COVID-19 care protocol. For them, COVID-19 was among many illnesses like measles, pox, and anaemia that 'Devi (ancestorial spirit) creates once every few years to punish the humans' if they fall short in the appeasement. According to Suresh Mandavi, a youth shaman, the conflict and the violence of the last two decades have caused an imbalance in the Adivasi cosmos. Due to displacements, the village elders could not offer any sacrifices to the guarding deities who resided at the borders of their respective villages, and the deities were left unsatisfied for a long period. These are also the deities responsible for protecting the villagers by restricting any evils from entering. In anger, the deity caused different illnesses among villagers. Although Suresh did not make this remark in the context of the COVID-19 pandemic, he believed that had the border deity been satisfied, she would have prevented 'Corona from coming into the Adivasi areas too'.

Although not a health emergency, this last vignette represents the Adivasi cosmology of preventive therapy and treatment. As against the biomedical system's individualistic approach, appeasing the deity for the physical well-being of the entire community presents a holistic approach to Indigenous healing practices. The already existing discriminatory attitude of the biomedical system in creating a forced separation between Indigenous healing practices and health centres was furthered by the preventative protocols prescribed and implemented during the COVID-19 pandemic. The scepticism among the Adivasi communities was a result of historical discrimination practised by the health practitioners who, despite their well-meaning intentions, ended up devaluing the Indigenous knowledge systems. While the ritual of appeasement may only be symbolic, the increased practices of these rituals and the beliefs of Adivasi youth in these systems indicate an increasing gap between the biomedical and Indigenous knowledge systems, which worsened during the COVID-19 pandemic.

4.9 Conclusion

The Adivasi community could not resist the vaccination drive for long as the administration took many coercive and persuasive measures to ensure that the vaccine was administered across the Adivasi areas. Among the persuasive measures, awareness camps were held and visual-aid messages about the vaccine were circulated over mobile applications like WhatsApp. Coercive measures were taken through restrictions such as withholding government employees' salaries and curtailing subsidized food provisions under the public distribution system and the National Food Security Scheme (PDS-NFSA).[61] The Adivasi youths who worked in the government sector were mandated to get vaccinations. Failing them, they could face disciplinary action, including loss of wages. For the community members not part of government services, a COVID-19 vaccine certificate was mandatory for them to collect their monthly provisions of subsidized food grains under the PDS-NFSA scheme. Despite these restrictions, the Adivasi communities' reluctance to vaccination is a complex response to the medical management of the pandemic.

Based on contrasting ethnographic vignettes, this chapter complicates the understanding of crisis management during the COVID-19 pandemic in South Chhattisgarh. I show that the Adivasi community's multifaceted response towards COVID-19 and other illnesses is rooted in onto-epistemological differences in the presence of parallel and competing medical systems. On the one hand, their experiences of modern biomedical systems are of historical systemic and social neglect and discrimination. I argue that the resulting health disparities are experienced as a continuum of violence.

On the other hand, the chapter also analyses Indigenous medical systems and communities' strong belief in traditional healing. I show that this parallel healing system offers a continuum of care. The Adivasi community, especially the youth in the movement against militarization, takes up healthcare as a collective responsibility by training in and administering aids in illnesses like malaria, common flu, and others. The elders engaged in the appeasement ceremony respond to illness by engaging in the Indigenous belief systems. In both these situations, the community response to the pandemic and other illnesses are illustrious of intertwined connections of care and violence. This interconnection between care and violence emerges from the 'interrelations and disjuncture of state programs'.[62]

Notes

1 There were multiple reports and news of fake news and misinformation about COVID-19 infection and vaccination being circulated in the world.

Tony Romm, Fake cures and other coronavirus conspiracy theories are flooding WhatsApp, leaving governments and users with a 'sense of panic,' *The Washington Post*. 2020. Accessed 30 May 2023. www.washingtonpost.com/technology/2020/03/02/whatsapp-coronavirus-misinformation/.

In addition to worrying about facing fertility issues, rural residents in India feared adverse health conditions, including death. A survey conducted in 2021 in rural India found that 55% of the people were afraid of the vaccine.

Puja Changoiwala, In rural India, extreme WhatsApp hesitancy. 2022. Accessed 30 May 2023. https://undark.org/2022/04/26/in-rural-india-extreme-covid-vaccine-hesitancy/.

2 The Covid-19 pandemic and health inequalities, *Journal of Epidemiology and Community Health* (74) (2020): 964–68.

3 Swati Birla, and Kuver Sinha, The making of India's vaccine famine, *Spectre*, June 2021. Accessed 30 May 2023. https://spectrejournal.com/the-making-of-indias-vaccine-famine/.

4 Nancy Scheper-Hughes, and Philippe I. Bourgois, *Violence in War and Peace: An Anthology*, Malden, MA: Blackwell Publishing, 2004.

5 Nancy Scheper-Hughes, and Philippe I. Bourgois, *Violence in War and Peace: An Anthology*, Malden, MA: Blackwell Publishing, 2004: 2.

6 Pierre Bourdieu, and Loïc J. D. Wacquant, *An Invitation to Reflexive Sociology*, Chicago, IL: University of Chicago Press, 1992.

7 Paul Farme, An anthropology of structural violence, *Current Anthropology* 45 (3) (2004): 305–25.

8 Nancy Scheper-Hughe, *Death Without Weeping: The Violence of Everyday Life in Brazil*, Berkeley: University of California Press, 1992.

9 Scheper-Hughes, and Philippe Bourgois, *Violence in War and Peace*, 2.

10 Scheper-Hughes, and Philippe Bourgois, *Violence in War and Peace*, 2.

11 Scheper-Hughes, and Philippe Bourgois, *Violence in War and Peace*, 6.

12 Michael Taussig, Culture of terror—space of death. Roger casement's putumayo report and the explanation of torture, *Comparative Studies in Society and History* 26 (3) (1984): 467–97.

13 Michael Herzfeld, *The Social Production of Indifference*, 1st ed., Routledge, 1992.

14 Scheper-Hughes, *Death Without Weeping*, 216.

15 Akhil Gupta, *Red Tape : Bureaucracy, Structural Violence, and Poverty in India*, Durham, NC: Duke University Press, 2012.

16 Bourdieu, and Loïc J. D. Wacquant, *An Invitation to Reflexive Sociology*, 15.

17 Jodi Kim, Settler modernity, debt imperialism, and the necropolitics of the promise, in Jodi A. Byrd, Alyosha Goldstein, Jodi Melamed, and Chandan Reddy (eds.), *Social Text*, Duke University Press, 2018: 41–61.

18 Sarada Balagopalan, Neither suited for the home nor for the fields': Inclusion, formal schooling and the Adivasi child, *IDS Bulletin*, 34 (1) (2003): 55–62.

19 Ian Anderson, Bridget Robson, Michele Connolly, Fadwa Al-Yaman, Espen Bjertness, Alexandra King, and Michael Tynan, et al. Indigenous and tribal peoples' health (The Lancet—Lowitja Institute Global Collaboration): A population study, *The Lancet (British Edition)* 388 (1040) (2016): 131–57.

20 Yogeshwar Kalkonde, Chetanya Malik, Manveen Kaur, Uday Pando, Gangaram Paikra, and Yogesh Jain, Why are so many Indigenous Pando people dying? Using observations from Chhattisgarh, India, to conduct structural assessment and identify solutions, *Global Public Health* 18 (1) (2023): 2175014.

21 Bambra, Ford Riordan, and Mathews, *The Covid-19 Pandemic and Health Inequalities*, 964.
22 Bambra, Ford Riordan, and Mathews, *The Covid-19 Pandemic and Health Inequalities*, 965.
23 Ankita Meghani, Manjula Sharma, Tanya Singh, Sourav Ghosh Dastidar, Veena Dhawan, Natasha Kanagat, Anil Gupta, Anumegha Bhatnagar, Kapil Singh, and Jessica C. Shearer, et al., Enhancing Covid-19 vaccine uptake among tribal communities: A case study on program implementation experiences from Jharkhand and Chhattisgarh states, India, *Vaccines* 12 (5) (2024): 463.
24 Gita Gopinath, The great lockdown: Worst Economic downturn since the great depression, *IMF Blog*, 14 April 2020. Accessed 30 May 2023. www.imf.org/en/Blogs/Articles/2020/04/14/blog-weo-the-great-lockdown-worst-economic-downturn-since-the-great-depression.
25 Nandini Sundar, *Subalterns and Sovereigns: An Anthropological History of Bastar 1854–2006*, New Delhi: Oxford University Press, 2007.
26 Alpa Shah, *Nightmarch: Among India's Revolutionary Guerrillas*, London: Hurst Publishers, 2018.
27 Virginius Xaxa, Identity, power, and development: The Kondhs in Orissa, India, in Suzana Sawyer and Edmund Terence Gomez (eds.), *The Politics of Resource Extraction*, London: Palgrave Macmillan, 2012: 180–203. n.d.: 180.
28 Virginius Xaxa, Identity, power, and development: The Kondhs in Orissa, India, in Suzana Sawyer and Edmund Terence Gomez (eds.), *The Politics of Resource Extraction*, London: Palgrave Macmillan, 2012: 180.
29 Nightmarch Shah, 280.
30 Ramchandra Guha, Democracy and violence: In India and beyond, *Economic and Political Weekly* 48 (14) (2007).
31 Nandini Sundar, *Subalterns and Sovereigns: An Anthropological History of Bastar 1854–2006*, New Delhi: Oxford University Press, 2007.
32 Rashmi Kumari, Constructions and contestations of Indigenous girlhoods in residential schools in Central India, *Children's Geographies*, 20 (6) 2022: 832–44, 35.
33 Navlakha.
34 Nandini Sundar, *The Burning Forest: India's War in Bastar*, New Delhi: Juggernaut Books, 2016, 25.
35 Accessed 30 May 2023. https://crpf.gov.in/org-structure-chhattisgarh-sector.htm, https://ommcomnews.com/india-news/crpf-to-set-up-more-forward-operating-bases-in-maoist-hit-areas-soon.
36 Accessed 30 May 2023. https://crpf.gov.in/org-structure-chhattisgarh-sector.htm, https://ommcomnews.com/india-news/crpf-to-set-up-more-forward-operating-bases-in-maoist-hit-areas-soon.
37 Accessed 30 May 2023. https://timesofindia.indiatimes.com/city/raipur/health-min-4-docs-suspended-for-corruption-during-covid/articleshow/98956488.cms.
38 Ashutosh Bharadwaj, *The Death Script: Dreams and Delusions in Naxal Country*, New Delhi: Harper Collins, 2020.
39 Accessed 30 May 2023. https://globalfreedomofexpression.columbia.edu/cases/binayak-sen-v-chhatisgarh/.
40 Accessed 30 May 2023. https://timesofindia.indiatimes.com/india/no-ban-on-medical-ngo-chhattisgarh/articleshow/2274666.cms.
41 Dilip D'Souza, *The Curious Case of Binayak Sen*, Mumbai: Harper Collins Publishers India, 2012.
42 *The Lancet–Lowitja Report*, 140.
43 Angeline Jeyakumar, Devishree Dunna, and Mitravinda Aneesh, Loss of livelihood, wages, and employment during the Covid-19 pandemic in selected districts

of Chhattisgarh in India, and its impact on food insecurity and hunger, *Front Public Health*, May 2022, 6 (10).
44 Ankita Meghani, Manjula Sharma, Tanya Singh, Sourav Ghosh Dastidar, Veena Dhawan, Natasha Kanagat, Anil Gupta, Anumegha Bhatnagar, Kapil Singh, and Jessica C. Shearer, et al., *Enhancing COVID-19 Vaccine Uptake among Tribal Communities*, 463.
45 Xaxa quoted in Amita Baviskar, The politics of being 'Indigenous', in *Indigeneity in India*, 1st ed., Routledge, 2006: 33–49, 45.
46 Kumari, Constructions and contestations of indigenous girlhoods in residential schools in Central India, 834.
47 Kumari, Constructions and contestations of indigenous girlhoods in residential schools in Central India, 834.
48 Helen Lambert, From 'medical men' to 'local health traditions: The secularisation of medicine in portrayals of health care in India, in *Situating Religion and Medicine in Asia*, Manchester: Manchester University Press, 2023: 198–218, 12.
49 Lambert, From 'medical men' to 'local health traditions', 203.
50 Lambert, From 'medical men' to 'local health traditions', 213.
51 Lambert, From 'medical men' to 'local health traditions', 210.
52 Rob Nixon, *Slow Violence and Environmentalism of the Poor*, Cambridge: Harvard University Press, 2013.
53 www.downtoearth.org.in/blog/mining/nowhere-to-go-how-exposure-to-coal-dust-has-impacted-lives-in-odisha-s-mining-villages-86888.
54 https://economictimes.indiatimes.com/news/politics-and-nation/fluoride-content-in-water-high-in-17-districts-of-chhattisgarh/articleshow/48198721.cms?from=mdr.
55 Sundar, The Burning Forest, 25.
56 Clara Han, *Life in Debt Times of Care and Violence in N eoliberal Chile*, Berkeley, Los Angeles, and London: University of California Press, 2012: 22.
57 Clara Han, *Life in Debt Times of Care and Violence in N eoliberal Chile*, Berkeley, Los Angeles, and London: University of California Press, 2012: 26.
58 Clara Han, *Life in Debt Times of Care and Violence in N eoliberal Chile*, Berkeley, Los Angeles, and London: University of California Press, 2012: 205.
59 Clara Han, *Life in Debt Times of Care and Violence in N eoliberal Chile*, Berkeley, Los Angeles, and London: University of California Press, 2012: 24–28.
60 Nandini Sundar, Divining evil: The state and witchcraft in Bastar, *Gender Technology and Development* 5 (2001): 425–48.
61 'The Public Distribution System (PDS) evolved as a system of management of scarcity through distribution of food grains at affordable prices. Over the years, PDS has become an important part of the government's policy for managing the country's food economy' (PDS et al.). https://nfsa.gov.in/portal/PDS_page#:~:text=PDS%20is%20operated%20under%20the,grains%20to%20the%20State%20Governments.
62 Han 2012, 25.

References

Balagopalan, S. 2003. Neither suited for the home nor for the fields': Inclusion, formal schooling and the adivasi child. *IDS Bulletin (Brighton. 1984)* 34 (1): 55–62.
Baviskar, A. 2006. The politics of being 'indigenous.' In Karlsson, B. G. and Subba, T. B. (eds.) *Indigeneity in India*. Routledge, 33–49.
Bharadwaj, A. 2020. *The Death Script: Dreams and Delusions in Naxal Country*. Delhi: Harper Collins.

Birla, S. and Sinha, K. 2021. The making of India's vaccine famine: Beyond the global North v. global South duality. *Spectre*. Accessed 30 May 2023. https://spectrejournal.com/the-making-of-indias-vaccine-famine/.

Bourdieu, P. and Wacquant, L. J. D. 1992. *An Invitation to Reflexive Sociology*. Chicago: University of Chicago Press.

Changoiwala, P. 2022. In rural India, extreme Covid vaccine hesitancy. *Undark*, 26 April. Accessed 1 March 2023. https://undark.org/2022/04/26/in-rural-india-extreme-covid-vaccine-hesitancy/.

Clare B., Riordan, R., Ford, J. and Mathews, F. 2020. The Covid-19 pandemic and health inequalities. *Journal of Epidemiology and Community Health* 74: 964–68.

D'Souza, D. 2012. *The Curious Case of Binayak Sen*. Mumbai: HarperCollins Publishers India.

The Economic Times. 2015. Fluoride content in water high in 17 districts of Chhattisgarh. *The Economic Times*, 24 July. Accessed 30 May 2023. https://economictimes.indiatimes.com/news/politics-and-nation/fluoride-content-in-water-high-in-17-districts-of-chhattisgarh/articleshow/48198721.cms?from=mdr.

Farmer, P. 2004. An anthropology of structural violence. *Current Anthropology* 45 (3): 305–25.

Gopinath, G. 2020. The great lockdown: Worst economic downturn since the great depression. *IMF Blog*, 14 April. Accessed 30 May 2023. https://www.imf.org/en/Blogs/Articles/2020/04/14/blog-weo-the-great-lockdown-worst-economic-downturn-since-the-great-depression.

Guha, R. 2007. Democracy and violence: In India and beyond. *Economic and Political Weekly* 48 (14).

Gupta, A. 2012. *Red Tape : Bureaucracy, Structural Violence, and Poverty in India*. Durham: Duke University Press.

Han, C. 2012. *Life in Debt Times of Care and Violence in Neoliberal Chile*. Berkeley, Los Angeles and London: University of California Press.

Herzfeld, M. 1992. *The Social Production of Indifference*. Routledge.

Ian, A., Robson, B., Connolly, M., Al-Yaman, F., Bjertness, E., King, A., Tynan, M., et al. 2016. Indigenous and tribal peoples' health (The Lancet–Lowitja Institute Global Collaboration): A population study. *The Lancet* 388 (1040): 131–57.

Jeyakumar, A., Devishree, D. and Mitravinda, A. 2022. Loss of livelihood, wages, and employment during the Covid-19 pandemic in selected districts of Chhattisgarh in India, and its impact on food insecurity and hunger. *Front Public Health* 10: 81077.

Kalkonde, Y., Malik, C. and Kaur, M. 2023. Why are so many indigenous pando people dying? Using observations from Chhattisgarh, India, to conduct structural assessment and identify solutions. *Global Public Health* 18 (1): 2175014.

Kim, J. 2018. Settler modernity, debt imperialism, and the necropolitics of the promise. In Goldstein, J. A., Melamed, J. A. and Reddy, C. B. (eds.) *Social Text*. Duke University Press, 41–61.

Kumari, R. 2022. Constructions and contestations of Indigenous girlhoods in residential schools in Central India. *Children's Geographies* 20 (3): 1–13.

Lambert, H. 2023. From 'medical men' to 'local health traditions': The secularisation of medicine in portrayals of health care in India. In Stanley-Baker, M. (ed.) *Situating Religion and Medicine in Asia*. Manchester: Manchester University Press, 198–218.

Meghani, A., Sharma, M., Singh, T., Dastidar, S. G., Dhawan, V., Kanagat, N., Gupta, A., Bhatnagar, A., Singh, K. and Shearer, J. C. 2024. Enhancing Covid-19 vaccine uptake among tribal communities: A case study on program implementation experiences from Jharkhand and Chhattisgarh States, India." *Vaccines* 12 (5): 463–68.

Mishra, P. P., Sravan, C. and Mishra, S. S. 2023. Nowhere to go: How exposure to coal dust has impacted lives in Odisha's mining villages. *DownToEarth,* 1 January. Accessed 30 May 2023. https://www.downtoearth.org.in/mining/nowhere-to-go-how-exposure-to-coal-dust-has-impacted-lives-in-odisha-s-mining-villages-86888.

Nixon, R. 2011. *Slow Violence and the Environmentalism of the Poor: An Interview with Rob Nixon*. Social Text Online (31 August, interview by Ashley Dawson).

Romm, T. 2020. Fake cures and other coronavirus conspiracy theories are flooding WhatsApp, leaving governments and users with a 'sense of panic'. *The Washington Post*, 2 March. Accessed 1 March 2023. https://www.washingtonpost.com/technology/2020/03/02/whatsapp-coronavirus-misinformation/.

Scheper-Hughes, N. 1992. *Death Without Weeping: The Violence of Everyday Life in Brazil*. Berkeley: University of California Press.

Scheper-Hughes, N. and Bourgois, P. I. 2004. *Violence in War and Peace: An Anthology*. Malden, MA: Blackwell Publishing.

Shah, A. 2019. *Nightmarch: Among India's Revolutionary Guerrillas*. London, Hurst and Chicago: Chicago University Press.

Sundar, N. 2001. Divining evil: The state and witchcraft in Bastar. *Gender Technology and Development* 5: 425–48.

Sundar, N. 2007. *Subalterns and Sovereigns: An Anthropological History of Bastar 1854-2006*. New Delhi: Oxford University Press.

Sundar, N. 2016. *The Burning Forest: India's War in Bastar*. New Delhi: Juggernaut Books.

Taussig, M. 1984. Culture of terror-space of death. Roger casement's Putumayo report and the explanation of torture. *Comparative Studies in Society and History* 26 (3): 467–97.

Times of India. 2023. Health min: 4 Docs suspended for corruption during Covid. 24 March. Accessed 30 May 2023. https://timesofindia.indiatimes.com/city/raipur/health-min-4-docs-suspended-for-corruption-during-covid/articleshow/98956488.cms.

Xaxa, V. 2012. Identity, power, and development: The Kondhs in Orissa, India. In Sawyer, S. and Gomez, E. (eds.) *The Politics of Resource Extraction: Indigenous Peoples, Multinational Corporations and the State*. Palgrave Macmillan, 180–203.

5 Intersections of COVID-19 Within Nomadic Lives

Nation-State Machinations and Pastoralism Within the Gujjar and Bakarwal Tribes of Jammu and Kashmir

Afreen Gani Faridi

The Himalayas of South Asia are home to many tribal communities; some of which practice transhumant pastoralism as a tool of social reproduction and production. The Gujjar and Bakarwal tribes of Jammu and Kashmir are one of the largest transhumant tribal groups which traverse across the Himalayas along with their flock. A historically marginalised tribe, the Gujjar-Bakarwals have been considered to have occupied the peripheries of the nation-state both literally and metaphorically. As a result, claims regarding their marginalised status, including by this author in the past (Faridi 2020, 227–66), have been often linked to their hesitance in engaging with contemporary mainstream institutions of governance and production. While the Indian government has promoted policy tools that enable tribal groups to represent their interests and become collaborators in the policymaking process, the tribal response to the state policy of marketisation & globalisation is nebulous (Agrawal 2005). The research contextualises the lived reality of the tribe in a period of paradigmatic political turn in the region—exhibited by the abrogation of Article 370—resulting in the restructuring of power. The institutional restructuring was made possible by an extension of a political shutdown into the pandemic lockdown which created an extended period of absence of local representation in government and policy-making.

As per the International Labour Organization (2020), pre-existing inequalities within tribal groups compounded the disparate impact of the pandemic on the marginalised groups. The report highlighted that the disparity in livelihood, health, and environment resulted in compounding vulnerabilities of food security, education, income sources, and chronic illnesses within tribal and migrant communities during the pandemic. A brief review of research undertaken on the impact of the COVID-19 pandemic on tribes in India reveals a history of institutional marginalisation acerbated by a lack of accountability and apathy of state institutions (Covid-19 and tribal communities: How state neglect increased marginalisation during the pandemic 2021). The Scheduled Tribes comprise 8 per cent of India's population, numbering 104 million individuals. As per government data, about 75 per cent of tribal villages were without access to healthcare, over 50 per cent had

DOI: 10.4324/9781003591641-8

no access to the Public Distribution System of food grains at a subsidised cost, and the same percentage applied to tribal villages without piped water (Sushmita and Harsha 2023; Saxena and Mohan 2021). While the vaccination drive was announced in India on January 6, 2021, vaccination coverage in tribal areas was significantly lower than that in other districts. Lack of health infrastructure and internet facilities impeded vaccination coverage within tribal regions of Jammu and Kashmir, such as the Doda district which is home to over ten thousand tribal nomads, and delayed it till the month of June. The delay in vaccination was not only a risk to the collective health of the community but also a hindrance to undertaking community activities, including seasonal migration, integral to the survival of the Gujjar-Bakarwal tribe (*The Indian Express* 2021).

The impact of COVID-19 on the Gujjar-Bakarwals has been registered across different parameters. Sharma (2021) locates the impact of the COVID-19 pandemic on the everyday activities of the pastoralists such as access to pasture, water resources, and interaction with members from other communities living in contiguous zones. Narratives at a micro-level have been recorded by Dar (2021) wherein the reader is made to dwell on the experiences of specific nomadic families who relegate the travails of migration, markets, struggles for access to livelihood and education, and emotional state of family members during the pandemic. Nisar and Nabi (2022) and Nag (2022) have situated the impact of the pandemic on accessibility of education and provided evidence of patterns of decreased promotion and retention of children in schools during the period of the pandemic. In addition, Rajput et al. (2022) and Majeed (2020) contribute to the discourse by specifying the challenges faced by Bakarwals due to delays in migration patterns during the pandemic. This chapter builds upon the claims made by these academics by locating the impact of COVID-19 on tribal pastoralists of Jammu and Kashmir, not as a reactionary phenomenon to a health epidemic but through an institutional lens which interrogates the complicity of state and society in using the pandemic for the needs of the hegemon.

As stated in the introduction to the book, the chapter urges the reader to look at the period of COVID-19 not just as a Zoonotic malaise (Ray and Bhattacharya 2023). To communities on the margins, the pandemic was an experience of institutional violence wherein state and social institutions, inhabited by the hegemon, were operationalised to further marginalise, dispossess, and exploit those vulnerable and without power. The aim of such an act is to strengthen and reify hierarchies of power to allow for a future of extractivism in a capitalist state. Such extractivism is only possible with an increasingly disproportionate wielding of power between the marginalised tribes and occupants of state power, actuated through the weakening of political rights and means of sustenance.

In undertaking an exploratory analysis of the changing realities in this frontier region of the Himalayas, this chapter shall reveal the technologies and instruments employed to affect an expansion of the 'modern' state and market into the 'traditional' sites of production and social reproduction of the Gujjar-Bakarwal community. The thematic analysis shall direct the reader to the deployment of identity narratives in re-shaping communities and the use of sectarian technologies to catalyse a shift away from their transhumant natures.

It is imperative to have a critical framework which contextualises the historic and contemporary political realities of the region of Jammu and Kashmir. The region bears the burden of conflicts arising from contested nation-state claim-making, displacement and forced demographic change through genocide, and questions of self-determination through a promise of a referendum (Noorani 2014; Naqvi 2016; Tripathi 2020). It is in this context that the Gujjar-Bakarwal tribe has negotiated its existence and lived reality with a recent paradigmatic change in the political and administrative structures of the region affecting its limited autonomy.

5.1 Traversing Across Tumultuous Terrains

The Himalayan state of Jammu and Kashmir recognised 12 Scheduled Tribes within its territory before being split in 2019. The tribal population comprised over 11 per cent of the total population in the region with over 140,000 individuals (Census 2011). The Gujjars bear the largest number of individuals (over 980,000) among all tribal groups in the region, followed by Bakarwals, the second largest tribal group in the region with over 110,000 individuals (Census 2011).

Often considered a 'twin tribe', the Gujjar and Bakarwals form one of the largest pastoral nomadic communities undertaking transhumance in the Himalayan region of the Indian subcontinent. As a transhumant population, work and materiality are collectively owned and the tribe's mode of production is intrinsically tied to nature—as they undertake seasonal migration with their flock for access to pastures. The community do not relate to the lands they access using private property norms—merely setting up shelters called *deras* close to pastoral lands in the upper reaches of the Himalayas in the summers and *kullas* during their seasonal migration to the foothills of Pir Panjal during winters. The Gujjar-Bakarwals are often attributed as 'custodians' (Ellis-Petersen and Qadri 2020) or 'guardians' (Faridi 2021) of the land as they keep tending to both forests and pastures while they traverse across it every year. The practice of migration is central to the 'social identity of the tribe with the word *Khanabadosh* or nomadism used as a social marker' (Faridi 2021). Furthermore, as followers of Islam, the transhumant nomadic nature of work bears religious sanctification as *Sunnah*—a practice upheld by the Last Prophet of Islam (Peace be upon Him). Hence, mobility in terms of space and time is crucial to contextualise the customs of the Gujjar-Bakarwal tribe, as their political, social, and economic decisions have been shaped by their constant ability to move to undertake livelihood through nomadic pastoralism (Faridi 2020). The innate relation of the twin tribes with nature and mobility can be witnessed in the translations of the community names. The title 'Bakarwal' comes from two words *bakra*—goats and *wal*—the one who rears (Sofi 2013); while 'Gujjar' has multiple claims of origin which refer to locations in Central Asia—highlighting the historical spatial mobility undertaken by the tribe (Rahi 2011).

In a cruel state of affairs, the tribal members face the threat of climate change due to the anthropogenic activities of a neoliberal society. While researchers are locating the impact of climate change on the tribe, this research is the first part of exploring the possibility of a 'metabolic rift' (Foster 1999) occurring within the tribe itself and the factors contributing to it. Set against the changed federal structure and state policy, stormy political climate and new policy regimes in Jammu and Kashmir, the research locates the shifts in the nature of labour within the tribe and the factors contributing to the change.

5.2 Demystifying Change in Production

Through the analysis of ethnographic studies on tribes, one realises the creation of a paradox between the preservation of tribal customs and practices on the one hand and the need for 'development' on the other. Despite the changing dimensions of the tribal ethnographic work, one witnesses the consistent presence of an 'endism' debate accompanying such analysis (Humphrey and Sneath 1999). The 'end of nomadism' points to significant changes in pastoral practices when directed by the modernisation paradigm implemented by the state (Brower and Johnston 2007). Such works depict tribal societies as antagonistic to the institutions of the nation-state; existing only in peripheries owing to spatial and political isolation as a result of internal decision-making.

Developmental discourses based on rational law, scientific agriculture, and commercialisation have acted as tools for extraction. This resulted in the reification of the peripheralised position of tribes with respect to the nation-state, especially one based on a centralised power delivery (Doolittle 2003). It is the contention of this research that the destitution of tribal societies in India through an analysis of tribal policies, programmes, and research based on 'exclusionary' politics is simplistic and misleading. The Indian State has promoted policy tools that enable such groups to represent their interests and become collaborators in the policymaking process; however, its policies of market orientation and globalisation have burdened pastoralists through privatisation and commercialisation of community-regulated resources (Agrawal 2005).

The chapter locates technologies employed by contemporary hegemonic institutions namely the state, market, and society—to assimilate and peripheralise the Gujjar-Bakarwal community within its zones of extractive exploitation. The technologies should be contextualised against 'adverse inclusion' (Nathan and Xaxa 2012) and 'biopower' (Foucault in Taylor 2010, 41–54) as a framework to determine the transformation in spatial mobility and ownership amongst the Gujjar-Bakarwal tribe in the 'modern' nation-state and the predominant market system. The author locates the positionality of the tribal community by analysing governmentality (Foucault in Downing 2008) in the region of Jammu and Kashmir using eco-materialist (Foster 2000) perspectives. The framework allows for an analysis which demystifies the technologies of dispossession and sedentarisation of tribal communities for inclusion in hegemonic institutions of extractive nature.

5.3 Technologies of Dispossession and Rifts in Ecological Labour

Bower and Johnston highlighted the role of geographical isolation in aiding communities to avoid cultural assimilation. Such a setting allowed for gradual adaptation to change across multiple generations and provided the possibility of 'allowing the old ways to coexist with or modulate new ways' (Bower and Johnston 2007, 11). Furthermore, cultural segregation through the selective implementation of new values was employed by native communities in response to new interactions. However, in contemporary times, the process of imperialism (Sen and Marcuzzo 2018) in South Asia using economic and political tools has overwhelmed the agency of communities to practice isolation and selective engagement with alien values—leaving no space for 'gradual accommodation of historic episodes of culturally transforming invasions' (Bower and Johnston 2007, 13; Kreutzmann 2012). This section locates existing technologies being employed by hegemonic groups in Jammu and Kashmir and their impact on the lived realities of Gujjar and Bakarwals.

5.4 Identity Formation for Political Contestation

Ghazala Jamil, in her book *Accumulation by Segregation* (2017), has highlighted the issue of solely considering the Muslim question in India through the parochial lens of identity defined by the 'other'. Extending the argument of Harvey (1976), Jamil posits the importance of viewing the social aspect of spaces by employing spatiality and positionality as a tool of segregation and capitalist accumulation in urban spaces. The historical positionality of the Gujjar-Bakarwals is moulded by a bloodied past having faced genocide in October 1947 enacted by the Dogra Rule in the Jammu region with the complicity of the Rashtriya Swayamsevak Sangh (Snedden 2001).

A senior bureaucrat at the tribal department of Jammu and Kashmir narrated to this researcher the extent of the violence enacted by the British colonial regents in Jammu and Kashmir—the Dogra Rulers. As the bureaucrat recounted the obfuscated past of how demographic change was brutally enacted by the state in Jammu while partition politics were enacted in the region, merciless irony reared its head. One of the major sites of violence against the Gujjar-Bakarwal Muslim tribes emerged as the currently named

Gol Market in *Gandhi Nagar*—named after the one whom history deigns as one of the most non-violent person. Gandhi Nagar, now a posh upper-class residential area inhabited by the socially and economically privileged majority, was once a common habitation, pasture, and waterhole for the Buffaloes reared by the pastoral community. *Keeping aside the file he was handed over to sign and locking eyes with me, the bureaucrat spoke with a measured tone*, 'At the time of partition, the Dogra armed forces announced that they had arranged transportation, as safe passage, for the Muslim tribes folk in the region to go across the border to newly demarcated Pakistan. As the tribal members reached Gol Market, Dogra forces gunned down the pastoral families indiscriminately. It is claimed that bodies lay strewn in the street for more than three days. Some survivors hid underneath the bodies of their brethren, while others fled to the Raika forest in the hills bordering Jammu to the east; hiding for weeks without food, water or information about their families'.

This state-sponsored tribal massacre enforced one of the earliest spatial demographic reorganisations post-British colonial rule in India with estimates up to 237,000 Muslims being killed and nearly half a million forcibly displaced into Pakistan and its administered territories (Fareed 2017) from the plains of Jammu.

It was not until 1991 that the community was formally notified as a Scheduled Tribe in Jammu and Kashmir via the Constitution (Jammu and Kashmir) Scheduled Tribes Order, 1989 and the Constitution (Scheduled Tribes) Order (Amendment) Act, 1991. Furthermore, it took another decade for the members of the community to be officially enumerated in the Census (Suri and Raina 2016).

In a region still negotiating over the claims of political self-determination between the peoples of Jammu and Kashmir and the Indian State, the representation of Gujjar-Bakarwals in claim-making in the provincial legislature has been severely limited. The lack of serious participation in a region with limited autonomy in the past is also traced to the absence of affirmative action towards a political representation of Scheduled Tribes in Jammu and Kashmir's legislative assembly despite extending constitutional recognition in 1991. Unlike Article 332 of the Constitution of India, 1950, the Constitution of Jammu and Kashmir, 1956, only provided reservations for Scheduled Castes by Article 47. While the community leaders have demanded reservation for 16 seats out of 87 assembly seats in the state legislature, the state only provided for reservation in local bodies (*Panchayats*). Furthermore, in an increasingly neoliberal democratic state, eligibility for 'participative' citizenship requires commensurate ownership of private property. As a community which does not traditionally recognise private property, the pastoral nomads have been historically disenfranchised for not possessing documents recognised by the nation-state for being a 'permanent resident'[1] and avail policies of affirmative action (Faridi 2020). The urgent need for land ownership in a private property regime can be seen with Gujjars—a predominantly 'settled' community—electing nine representatives for the first time in the 2014 Jammu and Kashmir legislative assembly elections, while none from the nomadic Bakarwal group have been elected till now. Until now, no woman representative has been elected from either community (Bhat and Gulzar 2019).

Purporting claims of benevolence, especially that of tribal welfare, on August 5, 2019, the Union government of India abrogated Article 370 and undertook a unilateral revocation of the limited autonomy of Jammu and Kashmir (Buchanan 2019). The abrogation was followed by the usurpation of the notion of 'permanent residents'—entrusted with the provincial government—with the new 'domicile' rules[2] controlled by the Union Government. These domicile rules have been enforced under the Governor's Rule during a period when the provincial legislative assembly and government lay dissolved (and continue to remain so as this piece is being written). The new regulations allow non-natives to claim local resources through economic and political bargaining with the intent to affect demographic shifts in the region. Reports estimate that up to 25,000 people have been extended the right to own property and government jobs (Kashmir Muslims fear demographic shift as thousands get residency n.d.). The Governor's recent announcement of promising land to 200,000 homeless has been challenged by major political parties in the region on similar lines (Land for homeless in J&K: Mehbooba Mufti claims attempt to change demographics 2023). These demographic changes have far-reaching outcomes politically with economically and socially powerful non-locals—who had emigrated to Jammu and Kashmir for employment—now being included in voter rolls and possessing the ability to bargain public resource allocation further away from tribal communities to urban settlements where ethnic hegemons dwell. The inclusion of non-native 'homeless' would also seek to overwhelm the political aims of local voters using brute numbers as a majoritarian democratic battering ram.

The political project post-abrogation includes 'delimitation' of electoral constituencies which seeks to reshape the Muslim majority character of the state (Tripathi 2020), to which the Gujjar and Bakarwals belong, by relegating them to a minority populace for electoral gains. The Delimitation Commission undertook a process to redraw the Union Territory of Jammu and Kashmir's assembly constituencies—which is solely undertaken by the Election Commission in the rest of the country. Consequently, the Hindu majority Jammu region gained six assembly seats while the Muslim majority Kashmir gained only one (Delimitation panel order redraws assembly seats map, Jammu gains weight, Kashmir loses 2022). The process of delimitation undertakes gerrymandering while redrawing political boundaries in the tribal-dominated Pir Panjal region—which played a decisive role in previous provincial assembly elections. For example, the Anantnag Lok Sabha constituency in the Kashmir region had been redrawn to include Pir Panjal and Chenab—an area separated from Kashmir by the Pir Panjal Range. The move only seeks to equalise the weight of the Jammu region in Lok Sabha when compared to Muslim-majority Kashmir while defying the administrative and geographic logic of the exercise. Optimistically, the exercise marks the creation of nine reserved assembly seats for Scheduled Tribes (Ali 2022); however, the inclusion of 'Paharis' in the Scheduled Tribes list only dilutes the claims of the Gujjar-Bakarwal tribe. The latter community launched a state-wide protest named 'Tribal Bachaho March' (Save the Tribals) (J&K: 'Tribals Bachao' protest intensifies over govt, move to declare upper castes as ST 2022) against such a measure of including the Pahari community in the Scheduled Tribes list. The Pahari categorisation is essentially linguistic and its members are ascribed as belonging to upper castes—from various privileged castes and religions—who have had greater administrative and economic control in Pir Panjal (Ayoub 2022). Such a tactic depicts the Union's intent of creating fissures in tribal areas—political and economic—to weaken the collective bargaining power of communities on the peripheries. These methods of erasure and redrawing past constituencies in tribal regions effectively seek to enclose, segregate, and sedentarise the community to vote and elect their representatives from deemed 'tribal areas' while fomenting intra-regional social conflicts in the region. Post-abrogation depicts an actuation of governmentality in the name of tribal emancipation which in reality weakens their bargaining power and claim-making.

Even as the majoritarian state co-opts tribal aspirations, the denial of belongingness continues to plague the community after the abrogation of Article 370 and the imposition of 'Akhand Bharat'. Two years after the dismantling of the autonomous federal structure, this researcher visited the highland pastures of Bhaderwah in Padri, bordering the state of Himachal. The region reeled under a curfew due to Islamophobic comments made by a member of the ruling party in India (Reuters 2022), with only selective mobility allowed. The pastures and traditional dwellings of the tribal community lay the end of the developmental state—the electric and mobile infrastructure halting three hundred meters before the tribal dwellings—where the government-established tourist zone ended. The community 'lambardar' (leader) met this researcher in a dark mud-lined *dera* (traditional dwelling) with old wooden beams bearing the weight of memories and aspirations while supporting the soot-blackened roof. Due to the extreme unseasonal rain and snow, and signs of changing weather patterns, the *dera* served as a safe space for all. The community members were forced to cook inside and share the shelter with their herd of milch animals. After enquiring about the reason for not having a separate shelter, the *lambardar* explained the futility of erecting new temporary shelters for the growing flock—human and non-human—as the local administration constantly demolished them. He said, 'Being neither Kashmiris nor *Pahadis*, we are looked at suspiciously as non-natives and encroachers. Our nomadic mode of livelihood is used as a justification for delegitimising our history of being traditional dwellers in this pasture across three generations'.

It is pertinent that the community found no local support even as land tenancy laws were enacted in the region, via the Forest Rights Act, due to identity politics in the region. The refusal of the local hegemonic community—both *Pahadi* and Kashmiri—to acknowledge their belongingness made it easy to enforce administrative bias and apathy. Even as the tribal folks occupied the commons since before the contested accession of the region to the Indian State, they never were legally recognised as its 'permanent residents'.

5.5 Immobilising Nomadism

Contemporary institutions affecting the mode of production have been gradually creeping into the spheres of tribal existence. As the Gujjar-Bakarwals undertook the process of carving spaces for subsistence within the ever-expanding locus of the nation-state, the assimilative nature of the hegemonic institutions towards these marginal communities has been adverse. Even as the community traverses into urban agglomerations during their migration, where power centres reside, the response at these sites of power has become increasingly maleficent. The response by hegemons has been primarily to ensure precarity and adversity within marginal communities accessing urban spheres in order to ensure maximum extraction, exploitation, and status-quo of disparity across social groups. With mobility as the central tenant for ensuring sustenance within transhumance, the imposition of immobility upon the Gujjar-Bakarwal tribe has been earnestly enforced as they access spaces governed by contemporary social and administrative institutions. The duress faced by these nomads in accessing pastures due to land fragmentation through international border-making is being further aggravated by the creation of internal administrative borders. This was seen after the erstwhile state of Jammu and Kashmir was split into two Union Territories of Jammu and Kashmir and Ladakh along ethnic lines after the ratification of the Jammu and Kashmir Reorganisation Act, 2019.

Decentralisation of systemic violence using informal power structures within the society has become an important tool for alienating and dispossessing Muslim minorities in an ethnonationalist notion of unified India. Using sectarianism in an era of authoritarian populism, Hindutva politics pushes the narrative of a homogenised culture as a requisite for 'Akhand Bharat'—anything not compatible with its parochial notion is relegated as the 'racialised other' and divested of rights to participation in its version of populism (Natrajan 2022). As a tribe practising Islam, the Gujjar-Bakarwal tribe during their journey into the Hindu-dominated Jammu region have faced multiple assaults by Hindutva terrorists targeting their livelihood and bodies based on exclusionary notions of identity. The culture and practices of the tribe have been stereotyped and demonised as inimical to the definition of 'Akhand Bharat' based on fanatic Hindutva values. The violence wrought by the hegemonic social groups on the minorities bears impunity and sanction by former's representatives within the government. Since 2014, ethnonational and sectarian politics implemented in Jammu and Kashmir have made Gujjar-Bakarwals its soft target and caused severe socioeconomic losses within the community. Inspired by Savarkar's articulation of rape as a political tool (Ashraf 2016), the bodies of the Gujjar-Bakarwal pastoralists became targets of sectarian violence—including sexual assault (Faridi 2020). Such violence by Hindutva non-state actors aims to impede the access of Muslim nomads to unsown farmlands and pastures in the plains of Jammu during the winters. While taking it upon themselves to enforce cow-protection laws,[3] cow vigilantes or 'Gau Rakshaks' attack the nomadic pastoralists during migration over accusations of cattle smuggling and consumption (Rahi 2017). These non-state actors attack children, women, and the elderly to intimidate and instil fear among their victims (Chilling video seems to show how Jammu cow vigilantes brutally attacked a family of nomadic herders 2017). In 2018, a minor girl belonging to the Bakarwal tribe was subjected to a fatal sexual assault, with the convicted being a part of the state's police force and a retired government official (BBC News 2018). In response to the tribal community's call for justice, the upper-caste locals, of the village in Kathua district of Jammu, including elected representatives of the BJP in Jammu and Kashmir organised a public rally—'Hindu Ekta March' (United Hindus March)—in support of the accused (Ahmad 2018). The right-wing locals denied the nomadic community from burying their child in the local graveyard, where they had purchased a burial plot. The end goal of such violence is to dehumanise Muslims and to stop the nomadic community from settling in and practising their livelihood in Hindu-dominated zones—to snatch control of dairy and meat production from the Muslim pastoralists in Jammu and Kashmir.

The mobility of the tribes and their ability to undertake livelihood suffered greatly due to the political shutdown along with the pandemic lockdown (Firdous 2020). This has wrought nothing but vulnerability among the Gujjar-Bakarwals who undertook migration to and settled in the Jammu plains during the winter of 2019. The political shutdown post-abrogation of Article 370 was so sudden and secretive that there was no possibility of preparedness. The subsequent economic blockade and shutdown of dairy and meat markets rendered the community unable to trade with the wool sellers and butchers in the Jammu region. Facing severe financial losses due to the lockdown imposed after the abrogation of Article 370 in August 2019, the community was left stranded in the Jammu region late into the summer of 2020 (Khuehami 2022).

An amalgamation of Islamophobia and inconsistent government orders indiscriminately suspending mobility during the pandemic acted as the final nail in the coffin for the Gujjar-Bakarwal community (Firdous 2020). In a region palpating with Islamophobia, the Corona Jihad narrative in the bigoted media found its way to Jammu where the Muslim nomads were ostracized from dairy markets of Jammu and denied access to farmlands and empty plots after being accused of being carriers of coronavirus (Kissu 2020).

On an overcast afternoon, while sipping tea at a family celebration in Ghaziabad, Jammu, this researcher sat with a gathering of prominent tribal members at the house of a popular radio, and now YouTube, host belonging to the tribal community. The courtyard looked towards the hillside dotted with single- and double-storeyed houses and haphazard housing colonies. The host sat broodingly, once the conversation turned to the past, even as celebratory music played in the background and hot tea cups of noon chai clinked against the saucers.

Looking away from the assembly towards the vista, the host said, 'These hills were once fields and pastures where the Gujjars would dwell in settlements. As the city expanded gradually after the clampdown on militancy, the settled Gujjar communities sold off their lands under the pressure of the market. The nomadic communities of Bakarwals would visit the pastures in these hills and the fields in [Hindu-dominated] Kathua region seasonally every winter. The two groups were dependent on each other—the Bakarwal's flock moved into the fallow field in the winter and rejuvenated it with organic excrement for the next sowing season while gaining access to local pasture and water bodies. Furthermore, the nomads would also buy grain and get *Chara* (fodder) in the form of plant residue after the harvest. After the rise of hate politics [Islamophobia], the Bakarwals had to face *azaab* (torment; referring to the Kathua rape case) and are not welcome in the region. They have to face the prospect of having to pay exorbitant rents for accessing and camping in fallow fields in the region of Kathua'.

The biopolitics of the government extended uniform measures to almost eight hundred thousand nomads stuck in the confines of rented parcels of land in Jammu until April of 2021. At the same time, the absence of medical assistance such as the provision of vaccination, sanitisers, and masks only left the community even more endangered in urban agglomerations with higher coronavirus incidence rates (PTI 2021). With increased heat, depletion of access to pastures, and no fodder for livestock due to the onset of sowing season the community faced material losses, worsened by the absence of safety nets such as free rations and job guarantee provided by the government under Public Distribution System and Employment Guarantee Act (Impact of Covid-19 outbreak and lock down measures on tribal and forest dwellers (Preliminary Assessment Report) n.d.). While the delay in opening up migratory routes for the community to travel to higher reaches as temperatures soared affected the Merino and local sheep with low tolerance of summer temperatures, the delay in issuance of 'Mattoos' or written permits for allowing the nomads to travel with milch animals only piled on to their woes.

In the Bathindi region of Jammu, crossing a row of under-construction houses, this researcher entered a demarcated plot of land (for residential construction) overshadowed by a skeleton of a high-rise apartment complex. In this spacious plot, a small temporary dwelling made of construction red brick and mud lay in the corner. A small tent made of bamboo sticks and stitched cement and sandbags lay to another side. Inside was a woman belonging to the Bakkarwal community, with her 4- or 5-year-old daughter. I asked if she was comfortable speaking to me or if I could come back later when her husband was around. I stood outside the threshold, as she narrated her experience from within. 'He has gone to do *dehari* (daily wage work) at a construction site and will not come back till it is dark. I am alone with my daughter. We lost all the flock during COVID-19 pandemic and relied on rations from locals, as no government aid came to us. The flock were dying due to the heat and we did not have resources to buy medicine or adequate fodder. So, we had to sell them quickly and incur a great loss due to the price offered. We will not rear sheep anymore, my husband will either move to Kashmir with the Darbar (J&K state administration moves seasonally between Jammu and Srinagar every season) and work in construction sites in Kashmir or be a herder for hire for someone. My daughter and I will not migrate anymore, I will stay back in a rented room and try and get my children admitted to the local school.'

This period from abrogation till after the COVID-19 pandemic saw the Gujjar-Bakarwals deal with higher costs of living, dwindling income sources, and postponement of transhumance. These led to a cascading impact on the livelihood and subsistence of the pastoralists with a reduction in the quality and number of the flock and decreased access to meat and dairy markets. The construction of internal frontiers (Natrajan 2022) through administrative policies and sectarian violence acted as a potent technology for divesting the Gujjar-Bakarwals of their ability to control their traditional mode of production and subsisting independently of the neoliberal market and state control.

5.6 From Sacred to Surplus: Adverse Inclusion in Hegemonic Institutions

While the Gujjar-Bakarwals look towards economic and social mobility through access to state services and markets, however, the response of the state and the market does not match their aspiration. The hegemonic institutions seek a transformation of traditional work into precarious work which can be mobilised for cheap extractivism while stripping the community of bargaining power. The nature of pastoral work at once is sedentarised but, at the same time, is left to be mobile in the form of migrant labour which could be utilised by infrastructural and mining projects. The sacred nature of nomadic work shall be stripped of its ecological concerns and be transformed into banal surplus work after the dispossession of Gujjars and Bakarwals from traditional land and epistemes. The transformation is actuated through devolution of institutional through ethnonationalist sectarian politics which mobilises identity politics against the Gujjars and Bakarwals using spatial locales (Pahari) and forward social groups besides Islamophobia.

We witness an expansion of the frontiers of a neoliberal state into the traditional sites of pastoral existence without commensurate benefits accorded to the Gujjar-Bakarwal tribe or honouring of the claims made by the representatives of the state. This essay shall act as a segue to epistemic and materialist evictions faced by the nomadic pastoral tribe in Jammu and Kashmir as sites of 'metabolic rifts' (Foster 1999) and 'primitive accumulation (s)' (Thomson 1990) for colonial and capitalist considerations.

As I reminisce about the visit to the *dera* set against the slopes dotted by wildflowers in Padri, the image which comes to my mind is the word 'Welcome' painted, in white, on the foremost wooden beam supporting the roof. The word summarises the quintessential hospitable and undiscriminating characteristic of the community, even as the word lost all meaning when the time came for the hegemonic state and society to reciprocate.

Acknowledgement

Afreen Gani Faridi is a recipient of the Indian Council of Social Science Research (ICSSR) Doctoral Fellowship. His chapter is largely an outcome of his doctoral work sponsored by ICSSR. A portion of the work was possible as a result of the Rosa Luxemburg Stiftung short research grant extended via the Mahanirban Calcutta Research Group. However, the responsibility for the facts stated, opinions expressed, and the conclusions drawn are entirely that of the author.

Notes

1 Article 35A of the Constitution of India extended to a 'permanent resident' of Jammu and Kashmir an exclusive right to acquire immovable property, jobs in public service, and educational scholarships. The law originates from the period of Dogra Rule protecting the economic rights of Kashmiri Pandits against 'Gair-Mulkies' or non-native migrants from Punjab (Kashmir Life 2019).
2 The domicile rules determine the eligibility for owning immovable private property and eligibility to apply for public service employment.
3 To understand the political economy of cow slaughter laws in India read Patel (2022) and Human Rights Watch Report on 'Violent Protection in India' 2019.

References

Agrawal, A. 2005. *Environmentality: Technologies of Government and the Making of Subjects*. Duke University Press. https://doi.org/10.1215/9780822386421.

Ahmad, M. 2018. BJP leader in front, Hindu Ekta Manch waves tricolour in support of rape accused in Jammu. *The Wire*, 17 February. https://thewire.in/politics/hindu-ekta-manch-bjp-protest-support-spo-arrested-rape-jammu.

Ali, J. 2022. J&K: Delimitation commission proposes sweeping changes to electoral map. *The Wire*, 6 February. https://thewire.in/politics/jammu-kashmir-delimitation-commission-sweeping-changes-electoral-map.

Ashraf, A. 2016. Reading Savarkar: How a Hindutva icon justified the idea of rape as a political tool. *Text. Scroll.In*, 28 May. http://scroll.in/article/808788/reading-savarkar-how-a-hindutva-icon-justified-the-idea-of-rape-as-a-political-tool.

Asifa Bano: The child rape and murder that has Kashmir on edge. 2018. *BBC News*, 11 April, sec. India. https://www.bbc.com/news/world-asia-india-43722714.

Ayoub, S. 2022. Will be a historical blunder if Jammu & Kashmir's Paharis get ST status. *The Quint*, 22 November. www.thequint.com/opinion/will-be-a-historical-blunder-if-jammu-kashmirs-paharis-get-st-status.

Bhat, J. A. and Gulzar, D. 2019. Political representation of Gujjar tribe of Jammu and Kashmir: An analytical study. *History Research Journal* 5 (4): 1448–54.

Brower, B. and Johnston, B. R., eds. 2007. *Disappearing Peoples? Indigenous Groups and Ethnic Minorities in South and Central Asia.* Left Coast Press.

Buchanan, K. 2019. FALQs: Article 370 and the removal of Jammu and Kashmir's special status | In custodia legis. *Webpage. The Library of Congress*, 3 October. https://doi.org/10/falqs-article-370-and-the-removal-of-jammu-and-kashmirs-special-status.

Chilling video seems to show how Jammu cow vigilantes brutally attacked a family of nomadic herders. 2017. *Scroll.In*, 23 April. https://scroll.in/article/835441/video-purporting-to-show-cow-vigilantes-attacking-nomadic-herders-in-jammu-emerges.

Covid-19 and tribal communities: How state neglect increased marginalisation during the pandemic. 2021. *Economic and Political Weekly*, 8 September. https://www.epw.in/engage/article/covid-19-and-tribal-communities-how-state-neglect.

Dar, U. A. 2021. Covid-19 pandemic in pastoral contexts: Reflection from the Northwest Himalayas. *The Eastern Anthropologist* 74 (2): 349–64.

Delimitation panel order redraws assembly seats map, Jammu gains weight, Kashmir loses. 2022. *The Wire*, 5 May. https://thewire.in/government/jk-delimitation-panel-signs-final-order-on-redrawing-assembly-seats.

Doolittle, A. 2003. Colliding discourses: Western land laws and native customary rights in North Borneo, 1881–1918. *Journal of Southeast Asian Studies* 34 (1): 97–126. https://www.jstor.org/stable/20072477.

Downing, L. 2008.Cambridge introductions to literature. In *The Cambridge Introduction to Michel Foucault*. Cambridge: Cambridge University Press. https://doi.org/10.1017/CBO9780511793240.

Ellis-Petersen, H. and Qadri, A. 2020. "They are custodians of the jungle": Anger as Kashmiri Nomads' homes destroyed. *The Guardian*, 4 December, sec. World News. https://www.theguardian.com/world/2020/dec/04/they-are-custodians-of-the-jungle-anger-as-kashmiri-nomads-homes-destroyed.

Fareed, R. 2017. The forgotten massacre that ignited the Kashmir dispute. *Aljazeera*, 6 November. https://www.aljazeera.com/news/2017/11/6/the-forgotten-massacre-that-ignited-the-kashmir-dispute.

Faridi, A. 2021. Unravelling the "PPP" model affecting nomadic pastoralists in Jammu & Kashmir'. *The Bastion* (*blog*), 9 August. https://thebastion.co.in/politics-and/environment/resource-management/unravelling-the-ppp-model-affecting-nomadic-pastoralists-in-jammu-kashmir/.

Faridi, A. G. 2020. Child labour in a pastoral tribe of Jammu and Kashmir: Impact of spatiality within a state of conflict. In Posso, A. (ed.) *Child Labor in the Developing World.* Singapore: Palgrave Macmillan, 227–66. https://doi.org/10.1007/978-981-15-3106-4_9.

Firdous, H. 2020. In Jammu and Kashmir, inconsistent lockdown rules have disrupted seasonal livestock migration. *Text. Scroll.In*, 4 May. https://scroll.in/article/960770/in-jammu-and-kashmir-inconsistent-lockdown-rules-have-disrupted-seasonal-livestock-migration.

Foster, J. B. 1999. Marx's theory of metabolic rift: Classical foundations for environmental sociology. *American Journal of Sociology* 105 (2): 366–405. https://doi.org/10.1086/210315.

Foster, J. B. 2000. *Marx's Ecology: Materialism and Nature.* New York: Monthly Review Press.

Government of India. 1950. The Constitution of India. https://www.constitutionofindia.net/constitution/constitution-of-india-1950/.

Government of India. 1989. The Constitution (Jammu and Kashmir) Scheduled Tribes Order, 1989. https://legislative.gov.in/document-category/volume-i-part-4/.

Government of India. 1991. The Constitution (Scheduled Tribes) Order (Amendment) Act. https://tribal.nic.in/downloads/CLM/CLM_1/17.pdf.

Government of India. 2019. The Jammu and Kashmir Reorganisation Act, 2019. Available at: https://igr.jk.gov.in/files/J&K%20Reorganisation%20Act,%202019.pdf [Accessed 22 Nov. 2024].

Government of Jammu and Kashmir. 1956. The Constitution of Jammu and Kashmir. https://jkdat.nic.in/pdf/Rules-Costitution-of-J&K.pdf.

Gujjars, Bakarwals await Covid-19 vaccination camps in J&K's Doda. 2021. *The Indian Express*, 6 June. https://indianexpress.com/article/cities/jammu/gujjars-bakarwals-await-covid-19-vaccination-camps-in-jks-doda-7346708/.

Harvey, D. 1976. Labor, capital, and class struggle around the built environment in advanced capitalist societies. *Politics & Society* 6 (3): 265–95. https://doi.org/10.1177/003232927600600301.

Humphrey, C. and Sneath, D. A. 1999. *The End of Nomadism? Society, State, and the Environment in Inner Asia*. Central Asia Book Series. Durham: Duke University Press.

Impact of Covid-19 outbreak and lock down measures on tribal and forest Dwellers (Preliminary Assessment Report). n.d. *Forest Rights Act*. https://www.fra.org.in/document/covid-19%20assessment%20report.pdf.

International Labour Organization. 2020. *Covid-19 and the World of Work: A Focus on Indigenous and Tribal Peoples*. https://www.ilo.org/publications/covid-19-and-world-work-focus-indigenous-and-tribal-peoples#:~:text=Drawing%20on%20new%20ILO%20data,COVID%2D19%20response%20and%20recovery.

Jamil, G. 2017. *Accumulation by Segregation: Muslim Localities in Delhi*. New Delhi: Oxford University Press.

J&K: "Tribals Bachao" protest intensifies over govt move to declare upper castes as ST. 2022. *Sabrang India*, 16 November. https://www.sabrangindia.in/article/jk-tribals-bachao-protest-intensifies-over-govt-move-declare-upper-castes-st.

Kashmir Muslims fear demographic shift as thousands get residency. n.d. *Al Jazeera*. Accessed 17 April 2023. https://www.aljazeera.com/news/2020/6/28/kashmir-muslims-fear-demographic-shift-as-thousands-get-residency.

Khuehami, N. 2022. J&K: Nomadic tribes suffer under permission Raj, corruption, and govt apathy. *NewsClick*, 27 May. https://www.newsclick.in/J%26K-Nomadic-Tribes-Suffer-Under-Permission-Raj-Corruption-Govt-Apathy.

Kissu, S. 2020. Covid-19: With no food, no mask, no sanitisers, Bakarwals stuck in Jammu delay migration. *NewsClick*, 20 April. https://www.newsclick.in/COVID-19-Jammu-Bakarwals-Nomadic-Community-Stuck-No-Masks-Coronavirus.

Kreutzmann, H., ed. 2012. Advances in Asian human-environmental research. In *Pastoral Practices in High Asia: Agency of 'Development' Effected by Modernisation, Resettlement and Transformation*. Dordrecht: Springer Netherlands. https://doi.org/10.1007/978-94-007-3846-1.

Land for homeless in J&K: Mehbooba Mufti claims attempt to change demographics. 2023. *The Indian Express*, 5 July. https://indianexpress.com/article/india/land-for-homeless-jk-mehbooba-mufti-change-demographics-8773739/.

Majeed, B. I. 2020. "We belong to nature and nature belongs to us": Ensuring transhumance during the Covid-19 pandemic. *Social Work With Groups* 45 (1): 32–38. https://doi.org/10.1080/01609513.2020.1843864.

Nag, S. 2022. *Impact of Covid 19 Pandemic on Tribal Students*. Jammu and Kashmir: Tribal Research Institute.

Naqvi, S. 2016. The killing fields of Jammu: How Muslims become a minority in the region. *Scroll.In*, 10 July. https://scroll.in/article/811468/the-killing-fields-of-jammu-when-it-was-muslims-who-were-eliminated.

Nathan, D. and Xaxa, V. 2012. *Social Exclusion and Adverse Inclusion: Development and Deprivation of Adivasis in India*. New Delhi: Oxford University Press.

Natrajan, B. 2022. Racialization and ethnicization: Hindutva hegemony and caste. *Ethnic and Racial Studies* 45 (2): 298–318. https://doi.org/10.1080/01419870.2021.1951318.

Nisar, F. and Nabi, H. 2022. After 3 Lockdowns and a Digital Divide, J&K's Tribal Children Unlikely to Return to School. [online] *The Wire*. Available at: https://thewire.in/education/after-3-lockdowns-and-a-digital-divide-jks-tribal-children-unlikely-to-return-to-school [Accessed 22 Nov. 2022].

Noorani, A. G. 2014. *Article 370: A Constitutional History of Jammu and Kashmir*. Oxford University Press India. https://books.google.co.in/books?id=6PQtDwAAQBAJ.

Patel, A. 2022. *Our Hindu Rashtra: What It Is. How We Got Here*. Gurgaon: Penguin Random House India Private Limited. https://books.google.co.in/books?id=fCyWEAAAQBAJ.

PTI. 2021. Gujjars, Bakarwals await Covid-19 vaccination camps in J&K's Doda. *The Indian Express*, 6 June. https://indianexpress.com/article/cities/jammu/gujjars-bakarwals-await-covid-19-vaccination-camps-in-jks-doda-7346708/.

Rahi, J. 2011. *The Gujjar Tribe of Jammu & Kashmir*. 1st ed. Gulshan Books.

Rahi, J. 2017. Why the attack on Kashmir's pastoralists is a big concern. *Down To Earth*, 25 April. https://www.downtoearth.org.in/blog/agriculture/threatening-a-centuries-old-tradition-57703.

Rajput, P., Jadhav, J. and Rahi, J. 2022. Sustaining seasonal migration: Struggles of Bakarwals amid the covid-19 pandemic. *Journal of Community Positive Practices* XXII (2).

Ray, A. S. and Bhattacharya, K. 2023. An overview on the zoonotic aspects of Covid-19. *Proceedings of the National Academy of Sciences, India. Section B*, 1–5 April. https://doi.org/10.1007/s40011-023-01445-8.

Registrar General and Census Commissioner of India. 2011. *Census of India*. Government of India.

Reuters. 2022. Nupur Sharma: India's BJP suspends official over comments about Prophet Mohammed. 6 June. https://edition.cnn.com/2022/06/06/asia/india-bjp-suspension-islam-comments-intl-hnk/index.html.

Saxena, A. and Mohan, S. B. 2021. Chapter three—the impact of food security disruption due to the Covid-19 pandemic on tribal people in India. In Cohen, M. J. (ed.) *Advances in Food Security and Sustainability*. Elsevier, 6: 65–81. https://doi.org/10.1016/bs.af2s.2021.07.006.

Sen, S. and Marcuzzo, M. C. 2018. *The Changing Face of Imperialism: Colonialism to Contemporary Capitalism*. Taylor & Francis. https://books.google.co.in/books?id=RBFFDwAAQBAJ.

Sharma, R. 2021. Covid-19 pandemic and Bakarwal pastoralists issues. *EPRA International Journal of Socio-Economic and Environmental Outlook* 8 (9). https://eprajournals.com/IJSA/article/5853.

Snedden, C. 2001. What happened to Muslims in Jammu? Local identity, '"the massacre" of 1947' and the roots of the "Kashmir problem". *South Asia: Journal of South Asian Studies* 24 (2): 111–34. https://doi.org/10.1080/00856400108723454.

Sofi, U. J. 2013. The sedentarization process of the transhumant Bakarwal tribals of the Jammu & Kashmir (India). *IOSR Journal of Humanities and Social Science* 11 (6): 63–67.

Suri, K. and Raina, P. 2016. A study of educational status of tribal Bakkarwal children of Kalakote block in Rajouri District of Jammu and Kashmir. *Asian Journal of Multidisciplinary Studies* 4 (11): 72–81.

Sushmita, and Harsha, S. 2023. *Fending for Themselves—Adivasis, Forest Dwelling Communities and the Devastating Second Wave of Covid-19*. The Hindu Centre for Politics and Public Policy. https://www.thehinducentre.com/the-arena/fending-for-themselves-adivasis-forest-dwelling-communities-and-the-devastating-second-wave-of-covid-19/article66640859.ece.

Taylor, C. 2010. Biopower. In Taylor, D. (ed.) *Michel Foucault: Key Concepts*. Acumen Publishing, 41–54. https://doi.org/10.1017/UPO9781844654734.004.

Thomson, R. 1990. Primitive capitalist accumulation. In Eatwell, J., Milgate, M. and Newman, P. (eds.) *Marxian Economics. The New Palgrave*. London: Palgrave Macmillan, 13–20. https://doi.org/10.1007/978-1-349-20572-1_47.

Tripathi, S. 2020. Throughout history, demographic changes to J&K have only deepened conflict. *The Wire*, 29 July. https://thewire.in/rights/jammu-kashmir-domicile-law-article-35a-permanent-resident.

Violent cow protection in India. 2019. *Human Rights Watch*, February. https://www.hrw.org/report/2019/02/19/violent-cow-protection-india/vigilante-groups-attack-minorities.

6 COVID-19 and the Indigenous Migrants' Question in Urban India

Aashish Xaxa

6.1 Introduction

The COVID-19 pandemic has emerged as one of the most severe global health crises, profoundly impacting economies and societies worldwide. Among the many affected groups, migrant workers in India have borne a disproportionate share of the burden. The sudden imposition of a nationwide lockdown on March 24, 2020, aimed at curbing the spread of the virus, left millions of migrant workers stranded in cities without jobs, income, or means of transportation to return to their native places. This humanitarian crisis has highlighted the deep-seated vulnerabilities of India's migrant workforce, particularly those hailing from tribal communities.

Tribal migrants, or Adivasis, constitute a significant segment of India's internal migrants. Originating mainly from Madhya Pradesh, Jharkhand, Chhattisgarh, Odisha, and the North Eastern regions, these workers migrate to urban centres for better livelihoods. Historically marginalised and socio-economically disadvantaged tribal communities face unique challenges that exacerbate their vulnerability during crises like the COVID-19 pandemic. The lockdown not only stripped them of their livelihoods but also exposed them to severe health risks and social stigmatisation.

The phenomenon of migration among tribal populations is deeply rooted in India's socio-economic fabric.[1] Historically, Adivasis have been compelled to migrate due to a combination of factors such as land alienation, lack of livelihood opportunities in their native regions, and displacement caused by industrial and infrastructural projects. Over the years, urban migration has become a survival strategy for many tribal families, offering them a chance to escape extreme poverty and access better educational and healthcare facilities.

However, the pandemic has thrown into sharp relief the precarious existence of these migrant workers. The sudden halt in economic activities left them jobless overnight, with many forced to undertake dangerous journeys back to their native villages on foot. The overcrowded and unsanitary living conditions in urban slums where many of these migrants reside further amplified their risk of contracting the virus. In their native villages, the return

DOI: 10.4324/9781003591641-9

of these migrants posed significant public health challenges, straining already fragile rural healthcare systems.

This chapter explores the multifaceted issues faced by tribal migrant workers in the context of the COVID-19 pandemic. It delves into the socio-economic conditions driving migration, the historical context of tribal displacement, and the impact of the lockdown on these communities. Additionally, it examines the governmental responses to the crisis and the efficacy of the measures implemented to support migrant workers. This chapter highlights the urgent need for inclusive public policies and robust social security measures to protect one of India's most vulnerable populations by providing a comprehensive analysis.

In doing so, this chapter aligns with the broader objectives of the volume in which it is published, which seeks to shed light on social justice issues and advocate for systemic reforms. The plight of tribal migrant workers during the COVID-19 pandemic underscores the necessity of rethinking urbanisation, migration policies, and labour rights in India, ensuring that the country's growth trajectory does not leave its marginalised communities behind.

6.2 Reading the Court and Legislation

The recent Supreme Court hearing on June 29, 2021, on the migrants' issue during the COVID-19 pandemic has thrown sharp light on what the apex court itself deems an "Unpardonable" apathy of the BJP central government. This chapter explores the impact of the lockdown on the tribal migrants in the country and seeks to explore their future in urban India.

The COVID-19 pandemic has unleashed multiple hardships upon the migrant workers of India. With the nationwide lockdown being announced on March 24, 2020, millions of migrant workers had to deal with the loss of employment and income, food shortages, and uncertainty about their future. Several thousands of them and their families went hungry. With no alternative to survival, they began walking back home, with no means of transport due to the lockdown, and with no help from either central or state government. A lot of migrant workers have been from tribal communities who belong to socio-economically and politically vulnerable groups in the country. This seminar will engage and address the issues and problems of tribal migrant workers from two different geographical regions of the country—Central India and the North East (NE). It will address the modalities of evolving social security and public policy measures, keeping them in mind.

As per the State of World Population Report (2016), more than half of the world's population lives in urban areas and the number is steadily growing every year.[2] India, where most of the population is still dependent on agriculture, is no exception to this trend. According to the census, the urbanisation level in India increased to 31.16 per cent in 2011 from 27.81 per cent in 2001. As seen in many Western countries, Urbanisation in India is mainly due to demographic explosion and poverty-induced rural-to-urban migration rather than an organic move towards an industrial society.

According to the State of World Population Report (2016), more than half of the world's population resides in urban areas, a steadily increasing figure. As per the 2011 Census, the level of urbanisation in India increased to 31.16 per cent from 27.81 per cent in 2001.[3] This urban growth is mainly due to demographic explosion and poverty-induced rural-to-urban migration rather than a natural shift towards an industrial society. The Economic Survey of India (2017) reports that approximately nine million people migrate inter-state annually.[4] The 2011 Census indicates that there are about 139 million internal migrants in India. The primary source states for migrants are Uttar Pradesh, Bihar, Madhya Pradesh, Jharkhand, Chhattisgarh, Punjab, Rajasthan, Uttarakhand, Jammu and Kashmir, and West Bengal, with Delhi, Maharashtra, Tamil Nadu, Gujarat, Andhra Pradesh, and Kerala as central destination states.

Tribal migrants from states like Madhya Pradesh and Rajasthan form the backbone of the construction workforce. In contrast, others from Bihar, Uttar Pradesh, and Odisha are involved in various low-wage, labour-intensive jobs. These workers, predominantly from marginalised communities, such as the Scheduled Castes (SCs) and Scheduled Tribes (STs), face additional layers of vulnerability in urban environments.

Most of them are recruited from villages through an elaborate network of contractors. Migrant workers end up being a vulnerable workforce that can be subjugated and disciplined quickly. The contract labour system and a loose monitoring and regulating state apparatus have helped strengthen these unfair models and practices in the migrant job market. In the unorganised sector, migrant workers regularly face conflicts and disputes at worksites. The common issues they face are non-payment of wages, physical abuse, accidents, and even death. The existing legal machinery is not sensitive to the nature of legal disputes in the unorganised sector. It has also been brought to light many times that several unorganised sector disputes never make their way to the labour courts or are kept languishing in courts for lack of proof thereof.

Indian cities are built on the hard labour and exploitation of migrant workers, but for some reason, they have never entered the consciousness of the architects, planners, corporations, middle class, etc.; instead, they are considered part of the problem in cities. The political class ignores them because they don't count as votes, especially in the case of inter-state migrants. Due to their mobile nature, they need help finding a place in the manifestos of trade unions. They spend their whole day on worksites and silently sneak into perilous shelters at night without the cities noticing them.

The origin of the virus is contested. However, the virus is thought to be natural and has an animal origin through a spill over infection. The first known human infections were in China. By December 2019, the spread of infection was almost entirely driven by human-to-human transmission, as confirmed by the WHO. The first case of COVID-19 in India was reported on January 30, 2020.

Most informal economy workers have little or no access to basic social security coverage. While India has made some progress in achieving a basic level of income security and medical care for all citizens, policymakers are facing a number of challenges, including closing the coverage gap, improving governance of social protection schemes, and creating the necessary fiscal space to fund social protection policies. The migrant labourers were returning to their home states from the states where they were stranded. During their travels, many labourers came in contact with infected workers. This led to a spike in the number of COVID-19-positive patients.

The health infrastructure in the villages could be improved. Inadequate staff has resulted in a shortfall of primary and community health centres. Sometimes, district hospitals are 200–300 km from the village. In these cases, there are no ambulances to ferry the people as the roads are poorly maintained, and people have to rely on their means of transport to get to the hospital. The number of tribal people below the poverty line is very high. This is compounded by the fact that malnutrition is very pronounced, coupled with a low mortality rate, body mass, stunted growth, and lack of potable water in the villages.

Migration among Adivasis is something that has been introduced previously. The emergence of the plantation economy in the British colonies had already drawn Chhotanagpur into its orbit as labour to be recruited from the region for plantation work in the West Indies and Mauritius (predominantly people from Eastern UP and Northern Bihar went and partly people from the Chhotanagpur area). The subsequent emergence of the plantation economy within India in the middle of the 19th century changed the pattern and route of population movement from the region. Indeed, the Chhotanagpur region provided the primary labour force for the plantation estates in Assam and Bengal all through the colonial period and continues to do so even today via the settled immigrant community. Both men and women were recruited as family units or as individuals.[5] They lived under an indenture or semi-indenture system, bounded within the confines of an estate and under constant surveillance. Wages were low, working and living conditions were inhuman, and working hours were inordinately long. Violence meted towards them was routine. Post-independence, there were some changes. Laws were enacted to protect and safeguard the interests of the plantation labour. They were also helped to unionise to further their interests. Yet they remain still the lowest-paid segment of the organised labour force. Unemployment is acute. Since the 1970s, there has been a surplus population in tea estates, but the work has been static as there has been no further growth of plantations. Hence, there is an absence of regular employment and a steady rise in unemployment.[6] Despite being part of the organised sector, their educational and health status is deplorable. Indeed, women from this sector have even begun to move to towns and cities in the region to work as domestic labour.

The other trajectory of population movement from the Chhotanagpur region in the post-independence era was to the Sundarbans in West Bengal and the Andaman and Nicobar Islands to reclaim land and forest and settle there as cultivators. Since the 1970s, seasonal migration from the region has begun. The movement is mainly during the winter for work in either agriculture or brick kilns or road repair and construction in border and hilly regions. After the 1990s, there was a significant shift to cities, not just towns in their state, but outside the state, because there were few opportunities in their state. They began to work as courier delivery people and guards. However, they were primarily employed as construction, domestic, and road construction workers. The earlier employment modes in brick kilns and border road construction also continued. However, with LPG, the marginalisation of land holdings, especially of small farmers and landless labourers, increased, forcing them to move out of their homes to seek livelihood.

Although historically, the predominant form of migration of the people from the region has been from rural to rural areas, in the post-independence era, there has also been a migration from rural to urban areas. The Chhotanagpur region was rapidly industrialised and urbanised in the post-independence era. While the fruits of such development did not go to the region's people, it did open up avenues, albeit limited, for the movement to urban centres mainly as unskilled or semi-skilled workers in industries and allied activities. The subsequent movement of people from the region into the metropolises has been made possible mainly due to the spread of education among these communities and the provision of employment reservations in government and semi-government institutions. In the past, the migration of people from the region to rural and urban settings was largely male-dominated. Women's movement was invariably tied to that of men as associated or dependent migration. Today, however, there is also a movement primarily of single, unmarried women, which is not tied to the movement of men.

In the case of the North East, historically and even in the post-colonial period, there was little migration of people from the North East to other parts of the country. Even if there was, it was mostly for education, and upon completion, they used to go back and get absorbed into state employment.[7] In the post-independence era, a lot of infrastructure construction took place in the NE, and it was operated by people who came from outside the NE, and it was not done by the Indigenous people from the NE. There has been comparatively less migration from NE to the rest of India until LPG. Comparatively, they have been better off than central Indian tribes. However, after LPG, the state employment in the NE was downsizing, forcing them to move out and seek employment opportunities outside. Even here, there is a distinction between hilly and plain people. Adivasis and Boro and Rabha tribals have been moving out to seek employment as labourers. Assamese cultivators and tribals living in lying areas have been moving to the plains because of floods, which have been encroaching on their lands. The rest of the NE tribes have been moving out to seek employment, mainly in the tertiary and hospitality sectors. They hardly go to the primary sector primarily due to social sector factors. They are found chiefly in malls, restaurants, urban areas, and the unorganised sector. That is why COVID-19 affected them because it got closed down. A lot of businesses worldwide are getting shut down. It impacts their branches in India including the hospitality sector, malls, restaurants and students.

The high mortality rate is due to a lack of medical facilities, doctors, distance, water, and poverty. Even if one person is affected, the chances of its spreading are very high. Livelihood is a big problem. They could be more skilled workers. Pressure on land and families will be more significant. It will affect diet. Another factor to be mentioned here is that the registration for NREGA needs to be higher because the land is owned by lineage or clan. The size of landlessness is relatively tiny, and migrants are often absorbed in agriculture. Health facilities are relatively better off, and the population is relatively smaller than the mainland; hence, there is little pressure, and the chances of their issues being addressed by the state are higher as their people also form the state. The CM of Mizoram praised Bihar for helping workers in Bahrain. This reflects the number of workers in Bihar.

Hemant has also shown great proactiveness in helping Jharkhand's migrants find their way home. Be it the first train or flight for migrant labourers, they found their way back home to Jharkhand. In an even more remarkable decision, he ignored the pressure of falling revenues and kept liquor shops shut for over two weeks more than most other states. In a first-of-its-kind evacuation of the migrant labourers, the Jharkhand Chief Minister booked a flight for the migrant labourers of the state stuck in Leh on Friday to bring them back to Ranchi.[8] The labourers were stranded in Leh following the lockdown and had requested to be brought back to their home state, understandably, after losing their work and finding it tough to survive there. The move comes a day after the apex court ruled that the state governments must ensure all help to migrant workers stranded in other states nationwide. With this move by Soren, Jharkhand becomes the first state to airlift 60 workers who will be brought from Batalik in Leh to Ranchi. On May 10, the workers reached out to the Chief Minister through Twitter, and the state government initiated a process to bring them back. Soren urged the Ladakh administration to assist them while the state arranged their return. The team mapped the stranded workers and booked a flight for the 60 migrants from the Dumka district stuck in Gorgodoh Village in Leh.

With support from the local administration, the workers were checked, thermal screened, and transported by the Border Roads Organisation (BRO) to Leh on Thursday. Sources said Soren personally monitored the whole exercise of airlifting the workers, which cost the government around Rs. 8

lakhs. He stood his ground for only sending about ten thousand labourers to work for the BRO in Ladakh, ensuring their safety, security, and well-being. The BRO and the Home Ministry had to agree to his terms.[9] Only weeks ago, Soren made arrangements for air tickets for many of these labourers stuck at inconvenient places in regions like J&K, Ladakh, and North East amid the raging pandemic. Most of these labourers are in demand by the BRO to make roads and other structures in Ladakh. They may have hardly been in the midst of their family when their requisition came from the BRO.

A little-known fact that should surprise people in authority is that the BRO prefers Jharkhand labourers for border road construction in high-altitude regions like Ladakh, Himachal Pradesh, Jammu and Kashmir, and Uttarakhand. They are solid and sturdy compared to their counterparts elsewhere and better acclimatise to tricky weather conditions. The Jharkhand Chief Minister has been at the forefront of raising the issues of the safe return of migrant workers to the state. Until now, around 4 lakhs of the total 7.5 lakh registered workers have been brought back to states by various means. Sources said the Soren government was working to airlift around 320 workers from the Andaman and Nicobar Islands soon. The work was on, the source added.

Jharkhand has tackled the migrant labour issue rather well. Adequate quarantine facilities were created at various places, and labourers complained about lessons. They behaved orderly and were left to go to their villages only after compulsory quarantine for two weeks. There are fewer reports of coronavirus-positive cases from villages in Jharkhand. These cases are mostly confined to cities and towns. What probably checked its spread was also alertness on the part of the villagers. Most roads going to villages from cities like the capital, Ranchi, were barricaded by villagers to prevent four-wheelers. As a result, the villages were saved. The villagers were also careful about the returning migrant labourers. An official said that they allowed only those with quarantine papers back to the town.

His proactiveness and clarity in decision-making have inspired great confidence in the residents of Jharkhand. Hemant Soren's listening ability is his most significant trait as a leader. In the case of Chhattisgarh, the Bhupesh Bagel government quarantined those who came through airports right from March and imposed social distancing very strictly.

"We have built 21,014 quarantine centres for migrant labourers and made it mandatory for those returning to Chhattisgarh to stay for 14 days in these centres. Most of these labourers were kept in quarantine centres near their villages only. Nearly 2.5 lakh labourers have already completed the prescribed duration of quarantine and have returned home. After the second lockdown, they started coming back."[10]

Nearly 3.13 lakh migrant labourers returned to Chhattisgarh and they were offered employment opportunities under MNREGA near their homes. They were allowed to register under MNREGA when they were in quarantine centres. In addition, the BPL families with ration cards were offered 105 kg of rice free as a three-month stock. Families who do not have ration cards were also offered 5 kg of rice. Migrant labourers were also provided with skill development training based on their choice. Another narrative below illustrates this:

> The government decided to give 70 kg rice to every ration card holder. But I was aware that many didn't have any card etc., so instructions were issued to give rice even to those who do not have ration card. I must tell you that the MGNREGA scheme proved very helpful in our mission to reach and help the poor. Right now, 22 lakh people are engaged through MGNREGA in my state. That is 24 percent of the total MGNREGA workforce in the country. That is how we provided money to a large chunk of our population in villages. Thirdly, Chhattisgarh is a forest and tribal dominated state. This is mohuwa and imliseason. We fixed mohwa-imli rate at Rs. 30 per kg. Earlier it was procured at the rate of Rs. 17 per kg. We have almost doubled the price. Similarly, we have issued new credit cards to 22.48 lakhs farmers. Our government also issued orders to all the factories not to do lay-offs. They were asked to provide food and lodging for the workers so that workers exodus don't take place. We ensured that our directives in this regard are enforced strictly.

During the lockdown, the Chhattisgarh government employed people in rural areas under MNREGA to save the rural economy. Presently, 23 lakh labourers, on average, work every day under various ongoing MNREGA jobs in our gram panchayats. There was a time in the second and third weeks of April when Chhattisgarh generated almost 90 per cent of the total MNREGA jobs in the country.

Apart from this, under the Farmer Insurance Scheme, Rs 900 crore has been transferred into farmers' bank accounts. Even during the lockdown, the government ensured that labourers in Chhattisgarh faced no shortage of employment opportunities. The RBI has also appreciated the steps taken in Chhattisgarh during the COVID-19 crisis. It has been stated in the RBI reports that the economic development rate of Chhattisgarh is better than that of many other developed states. During this time, forest produce collectors have also been given relief. The support price of *Mahua* flower was hiked from Rs 18 per kg to Rs 30 per kg. As many as 25 minor forest products are being procured at support prices in Chhattisgarh.

"We purchased minor forest produce worth more than Rs 18.63 crore, the highest in the country. We chalked out a multi-pronged strategy to help people experiencing poverty and implemented it strictly. It worked in our favour. Rajiv Gandhi Kisan Nyay Yojana is a small component of the original NYAY scheme, Rahul Gandhi's dream project. The theme is to transfer money into people's pockets directly. Under Rajiv Gandhi Kisan Nyay Yojna, Rs 5,750 crore will be transferred into the bank accounts of over 19 lakh farmers. The first instalment of Rs 1,500 crore under the scheme was transferred to farmers' banks. The amount will prove highly beneficial to farmers during this crisis period, helping them procure seeds, fertilisers, etc. Here I mention that earlier, we had made record procurement of 83 lakh metric tonnes of paddy, which has led to a significant improvement in our state's rural economy."

A quarantine centre with 700 beds was set up at the Sarusojai Sports Complex, and the government rented an apartment nearby, where at least 200 doctors can stay. Isolation ward of 200 beds at Sonapur Hospital, ICU ward of 30 beds at Gauhati Medical College and Hospital, 150 beds at Mahendra Mohan Choudhury Hospital, and 50 beds at Jorhat Medical College and Hospital were also set up by the government.

The government also established a fully functional, air-conditioned, 236-bedded COVID-19 unit at GMCH, including 50 ICUs and 186 wards.[11] The government also upgraded Jalukbari Ayurvedic College (Guwahati) into a full-fledged 110-bedded COVID-19 hospital. Quarantine wards with 1500 beds were also set up for Assam Police Personnel. 30 doctors and around 200 nurses were kept exclusively for the police personnel. Nearly 5 lakh people were screened across Assam, of which 36,818 passengers were screened at six airports in the state.

In the case of Meghalaya, the government increased its COVID-19 testing capacity to 400 per day by the end of May 2020 with the installation of a new Reverse Transcription Polymerase Chain Reaction (RT-PCR) machine at the North Eastern Indira Gandhi Regional Institute of Health and Medical Sciences (NEIGRIHMS). Those who came back to the state on Tuesday entered via the four designated checkpoints—ranchera in East Jaintia Hills, byrnie in Ri Bhoi, dainadubi in North Garo Hills, and Tikrikilla in West Garo Hills District. While several persons arranged their transportation, the Meghalaya government, in coordination with the Assam government, had arranged for buses to convey those stranded in Assam.

The anti-trafficking activist and founder of Impulse NGO Network Hasina Kharbhih planned to move the NGT to divert Rs 800 crores from the Meghalaya Environment Protection and Restoration fund that was supposed to be collected from coal mine owners towards a COVID-19 fund to help the labourers. From their preliminary assessment and mapping of existing active coal mines in the state, they estimated that there are 15,000 labourers—both migrants and locals—still working in coal mines.

"Meghalaya is unlike the rest of India, where thousands walk across state lines. With the prevailing insider-outsider politics, it's difficult for migrant labourers to do that here."

As mentioned before, around 92.37 per cent of the labour force in India is in the unorganised sector. Several schemes and programmes are in operation to provide social security benefits to these workers. The Unorganised Workers Social Security Act of 2008 is an umbrella act that addresses the welfare aspects of the unorganised sector. Aam Aadmi Bima Yojana provides life and disability coverage to all the rural landless households in the country. Under the National Old Age Pension Scheme, persons who are living Below the Poverty Line and are above the age of 65 are provided a pension. The government has enacted legislation to set up Five Labour Welfare Funds to provide social security, medical care, and other facilities to workers in the beedi industry and certain non-coal mines. The government started the co-contributory Pension Scheme—Swavalamban, in September 2010, where an unorganised sector employee contributing between Rs 1,000 and Rs 12,000 per annum for retirement savings is eligible to receive a matching contribution of Rs 1000 per annum from the government.

Since the lockdown, many questions have been raised about the welfare and the legal protection rights of migrant workers. The people working for the labour welfare have recalled the "Migrant Workers Protection Law of 1979" to regulate the employment and improve the working conditions of the migrant workers. However, the law is not strictly implemented. This law applies to all establishments employing five or more migrant workers from other states. In addition to this, this law is also applicable to contractors who have used five or more inter-state workers.

To address these issues, the government should implement targeted social security schemes for tribal migrants, improve healthcare infrastructure in rural areas, and ensure better labour law enforcement in urban settings. Establishments must be registered with the local authority while employing migrant workers. This means an establishment is prohibited from employing migrant workers from other states if they do not have a certificate from the concerned authority. The same law applies to contractors who use and deploy workers from one state to different states.

The law helps the migrants in the following ways:

- The registration of the establishments deploying migrant labour creates a system of accountability and acts as the first layer of formalising the utilisation of their labour.
- It also helps the government track the number of workers employed by establishments and provides a legal basis for improving the conditions of migrant workers.
- As per this law, the contractors deploying the migrant workers must provide terms and conditions of the recruitment to the workers. These are the remuneration payable, hours of work, fixation of wages, and other essential amenities.
- The wage rates, number of holidays, working hours, and other recruitment conditions for a migrant worker must be the same as those extended to other local workmen in the same establishment, provided that the nature of their work is the same.
- The wages of migrant workers must be at least those mentioned in the Minimum Wages Act.

Currently, there are 44 labour laws in the country. The central government wants these 44 laws to be coded under four laws—Wage Code, Industrial Safety and Welfare, Social Security, and Industrial Relations. The Occupational Safety, Health and Working Conditions Code, 2019, was passed in Lok Sabha on July 23, 2019. It was referred to the standing committee on October 9, 2019, and the standing committee made a report on February 11, 2020. The Code is still pending to be passed in Rajya Sabha. This Code repeals 13 of 44 labour laws related to safety, health, and working conditions. The Inter-State Migrant Workmen (Regulation of Employment and Conditions of Service) Act, 1979, is also included under this Code. These 13 laws include—the Factories Act, Mines Act, Dock Workers' Act, the Inter-State Migrant Workmen Act, and other enactments relating to those working in plantations, construction, cinema, beedi and cigarette manufacture, motor transport, and the media.

The new Code (2019) has similar provisions to the 1979 Act. It envisages the allowance of displacement and journey to inter-state migrant workers. However, the Centre of Indian Trade Unions (CITU) has highlighted that the 2019 Code and the 1979 Act must not be merged together and must be implemented strictly for improved conditions of migrant workers. Despite this act's existence, it has yet to be brought to work in the current situation.

However, if we contrast this with the ILO framework on migrant labourers, the difference is striking. The ILO Multilateral Framework on Labour Migration (2006) calls for the conclusion of social security agreements for the benefit of migrant workers. Social security agreements are treaties which coordinate the social security schemes of two or more countries to ensure the portability of social security entitlements. In some origin countries, social security schemes might be insufficiently developed, which is a problem for agreements that apply on a reciprocal basis:

- Social security schemes can also differ considerably— that is, disparity in the design and level of benefits (e.g. provident funds/social insurance schemes).
- Administrative capacity can be insufficient.
- Lack of willingness on the part of some countries to conclude agreements.

6.3 Conclusion

The COVID-19 pandemic has exposed the vulnerabilities of tribal migrant workers in urban India. While state governments have made efforts to support these workers, more comprehensive and inclusive policies that address their unique challenges are needed. This includes improving health infrastructure in rural areas, ensuring fair wages and safe working conditions, and providing social security coverage for all informal economy workers.

By highlighting the plight of tribal migrant workers and advocating for policy changes, this chapter aligns with broader discussions on social justice and equity in the volume it is part of. Addressing these issues is crucial for building a more inclusive and resilient urban India.

Notes

Primary Healthcare denotes the first level of contact between individuals and families with the health system. According to the Alma Ata Declaration of 1978, Primary Healthcare was to serve the community; it included care for mother and child, which included family planning, immunisation, prevention of locally endemic diseases, treatment of common diseases or injuries, provision of essential facilities, health education, provision of food and nutrition, and adequate supply of safe drinking water. In India, Primary Healthcare is provided through a network of sub-centres and Primary Health Centres in rural areas. In contrast, it is provided through Health posts and Family Welfare Centres in urban areas. The sub-centre comprises one auxiliary nurse, a midwife, and a multipurpose health worker. It serves a population of 5000 in plains and 3000 in hilly and tribal areas. The Primary Health Centre (PHC), staffed by a Medical Officer and other paramedical staff, serves a population of 30,000 in plains and 20,000 in hilly, tribal, and backward areas. Each PHC needs to supervise 6 sub-centres.

Secondary Healthcare

Secondary Healthcare is a second tier of the health system in which patients from Primary Healthcare are referred to specialists in higher hospitals for treatment. In India, the health centres for Secondary Healthcare include district hospitals and community health centres at the block level.

Tertiary Healthcare

Tertiary Healthcare refers to a third level of the health system, where specialised consultative care is provided, usually on primary and secondary medical care referrals. Specialised Intensive Care Units, advanced diagnostic support services, and specialised medical personnel are the critical features of Tertiary Healthcare. In India, under the public health system, tertiary care services are provided by medical colleges and advanced medical research institutes.

Notes

1 A. Sharma, Migration patterns and employment in Indi, *Journal of Migration Studies* (2020).
2 For further details, see United Nations Population Fund, UNFPA state of world population, 2016. Accessed 10 January 2024. www.unfpa.org/press/unfpa-state-world-population-2016.

3 Registrar General & Census Commissioner, India, *Census of India 2011*, New Delhi: Ministry of Home Affairs, Government of India, 2011.
4 Ministry of Finance, Government of India, *Economic Survey*, 2017.
5 S. Mukherjee, Colonial economy and migration: The Indian indentured labour in the Indian Ocean Region, *Economic and Political Weekly*, 2018.
6 National Sample Survey Office (NSSO), *Report on Employment and Unemployment*, 2017–18.
7 S. Baruah, *Migration and Development in Northeast India*, North Eastern Hill University, 2020.
8 Jharkhand Chief Minister Hemant Soren airlifts migrant workers from Leh, *Times Now News*. Accessed 30 January 2024. www.timesnownews.com/india/article/jharkhand-chief-minister-hemant-soren-airlifts-migrant-workers-from-leh/598568.
9 Migrant laborers, *News Abode*. Accessed 30 January 2024. https://newsabode.com/migrant-laborers/.
10 Poorly planned lockdown and unlock caused Covid-19 spike in Chhattisgarh, says CM Bhupesh Baghel, *Firstpost*. Accessed 30 January 2024. www.firstpost.com/india/poorly-planned-lockdown-and-unlock-caused-covid-19-spike-in-chhattisgarh-says-cm-bhupesh-baghel-8483781.html.
11 https://northeastlivetv.com/topnews/2-more-tests-covid-19-positive-in-assam/.

7 Mobile Theatre of Assam

The COVID-19 Pandemic, Challenges, and Responses

Rituparna Patgiri

7.1 Introduction

> 'Mobile theatre will not survive the test of time. It cannot stand the digital onslaught.'

I quote a celebrated playwright from Assam who told me very clearly that he does not see a bright future for Assam's unique theatrical tradition of mobile theatre during my fieldwork in 2019. This was in the backdrop of the growing popularity of digital forms of entertainment. As the COVID-19 pandemic hit the world in 2020, this prediction started looking more and more plausible. On 25 March 2020, a nationwide lockdown of 21 days was announced by the Indian Prime Minister Narendra Modi in an effort to prevent the spread of the COVID-19 virus. Similar to all other forms of performance-based activities, mobile theatre of Assam was also impacted. As more rounds of lockdowns were announced in 2020 and 2021, this particular theatrical practice was staring at an uncertain future. Stories of artists[1] leaving mobile theatre and choosing other forms of employment like selling vegetables and daily wage labour were making headlines in regional news (Kalita 2020; Barman 2022).

As I was consuming these news items, I was often thinking about what this particular playwright had told me in 2019. It was not an isolated view, but one that was shared by many dramatists and playwrights whom I had interviewed for my PhD fieldwork. It led me to wonder and ask the question that I never wanted to—is this the end of Assam's mobile theatre? I had never wanted to actually think about it because of several reasons. The first and most obvious is that as a daughter of a playwright myself, I had grown up watching a lot of mobile theatre, particularly in my childhood. Secondly, I have been researching and working on it for more than seven years and as such, there was an emotional affinity with both mobile theatre and the people who practice it. But with so much noise about how the pandemic was impacting it, there was no escape any more. There were journalists and others who often asked for my opinion considering my 'expertise.' As such, as a

DOI: 10.4324/9781003591641-10

researcher, I had to enter the conversation. This paper is a very small attempt at doing that.

I must admit that it has been very difficult for me to write this paper. One of the reasons is that I have been in the midst of several personal crises. But the major cause is that I am confronting an ethical dilemma—as an academic should I pontificate and write about the impact of the pandemic on mobile theatre when in reality people are suffering from its consequences? It has not been easy to juggle with this dilemma. Nonetheless, this is my humble attempt at bringing to light the way the pandemic and multiple lock downs have impacted Assam's mobile theatre.

Mobile theatre has been a major source of employment in rural Assam in the pre-pandemic years. However, the COVID-19 pandemic has disrupted their operation, and consequently there has been a massive job loss. As a significant part of Assam's cultural industry, it has informality in its employment structure. Therefore, the worst affected are the technical artists and workers with no support from either the owners of the theatre groups or the government. They do not earn a fixed salary every month and are dependent on contract-based work. Most of them were forced to shift to alternative employment opportunities, in either the farming or non-farming sector (Patgiri 2020).

This paper attempts to look at the impact of the COVID-19 pandemic on the mobile theatre of Assam. I argue that the impact is not just economic, but it has also influenced the cultural practice of mobile theatre. It also argues that the brunt of the adverse consequences of the pandemic has been borne by the technical artists and other workers involved in activities like cooking and cleaning. Most of them belong to the lower strata of society and are from rural Assam. The people who were most affected were at the margins of society—in terms of caste, class, and region. Thus, it is a crisis of marginality which has inter-relations with both poverty and social exclusion. By using a combination of interviews with people involved with mobile theatre and content analysis of newspaper reports, I try to explore this marginality. The closure of museums, galleries, cultural centres, theatres, and halls impacted the cultural industry but the influence was not homogeneous.

Performing arts was one of the sectors that faced the major brunt of the pandemic (Dinardi et al. 2023). The pandemic exacerbated long-standing issues of precarity and informality that have often plagued the performing arts (Comunian and Lauren 2020; Banks and O'Connor 2021; Jones 2022). There was a crisis of public space for performance-related activities (Khofifah et al. 2022). A critical transition occurred in activities related to theatre and live performance as they were compelled to shift online (Houlihan and Morris 2021). Similarly, performing arts across India have been pushed to the brink during the pandemic (Wadhwa and Kav 2021). In Assam, along with mobile theatres, mime and skit theatres also suffered (Patgiri 2021).

Readers then might be wondering why the story of mobile theatre should be told—what is so special about a form of theatre that it should be given academic space when almost all performance-based activities have suffered. At the outset, let me state that while many performing artists shifted to conducting online classes, workshops and performances, it is difficult to perform theatre online. This is especially true for mobile theatre which requires open space for a stage to be set up. It is also by definition a group-based activity. There is no possibility of private or intimate performances or online platforms to showcase theatre. Also, since the mobile theatre of Assam has a rural background, it is even more difficult to shift online. There is no luxury of uninterrupted electricity and internet connectivity as well.

In addition, there was little or no state support for mobile theatre. To cite one example, the government of Assam's report published in 2020 does not look into the impact of the pandemic on performing arts, including mobile theatre (SITA, Government of Assam 2020). This is even though Assam has a rich tradition of performing arts which includes folk practices like *Ojhapali, Dhuliya, Nisukoni Geet, Kushan Gaan, Bhari Gaan, Putala Naach, Bhaona, Ankiya Naat*, etc. There is also the presence of a vibrant theatrical culture and classical dance. Mobile theatre, however, is a popular form of entertainment which generates high revenues and acts as a source of employment. To provide more context, let me first state what mobile theatre and its importance in the context of Assam are.

7.2 Mobile Theatre: An Overview

7.2.1 History and Categorisation

Mobile theatre is a central part of the Assamese public sphere and public culture. It caters to a larger audience and is successful in the market (Ross 2017, 65). Mobile theatre groups (known as *Bhramyaman natak* in Assamese) comprise a combination of actors, singers, dancers, directors, action artists, make-up artists, workers, and the producer (Patgiri 2019). These theatre troops travel across the state performing their plays, carrying all the necessary equipment with them, ranging from stage material to props.

Mobile theatre is one of the most widespread forms of entertainment in Assam. Almost 150–160 mobile theatre groups have come into being in Assam since the first one was started in the 1920s. Before the COVID-19 pandemic hit the world, around 60 theatre groups were performing their plays in the state. These numbers keep changing as many groups close down and new ones start. What these approximate figures clearly show is the widespread popularity of mobile theatre in Assam. This popularity is also evident, as there are posters, hoardings, and signboards of various theatre groups all across the state.

Mobile theatre's existence in Assam is not recent. The *Sila Kalika Opera Party* and *Assam Kohinoor Opera Party*—the first mobile theatre-like groups—were founded and started by Brajanath Sarma in the 1920s in the Barpeta district of lower Assam. Assamese mobile theatre cannot be categorised as either classical or folk theatre. Although mobile theatre is not classical or folk theatre, it is also not modern Indian theatre in the conventional sense. Modern Indian theatre could not penetrate India's rural hinterlands as it was seen as too 'urban' and 'elite.' Neither did it use local languages (Awasthi and Schechner 1989, 68).

Mobile theatre in Assam, on the contrary, had begun in the rural context and increasingly spread to urban areas. It started in Pathshala, a town, about 110 kilometres from the city of Guwahati, the capital of Assam. In popular parlance, Pathshala is known as the 'Hollywood of Assam' or 'Natyagiri' because of the presence of the headquarters of a large number of mobile theatre parties in the town. Even though the *Assam Kohinoor Opera Party* did not last for long, the idea of mobile theatre had spread in Pathshala and neighbouring parts of lower Assam. On 2 October 1963, Achyut Lahkar, a pioneering figure in the history of mobile theatre in Assam, started the Nataraj theatre group inspired by Sarma's idea of the *Assam Kohinoor Opera Party*. The first play that was performed by Nataraj was *Bhogjora* in Pathshala's Hari Mandir (Talukdar *in* Das 2018, 112). Other theatre groups like Surdevi, Assam Star, Mukunda, Roopkonwar, Purbajyoti, Mancharoopa, Rupanjali, and Amar theatre also made their presence felt during this period. Consequently, Ratan Lahkar—Achyut Lahkar's nephew—began the Kohinoor theatre party in 1976.

While Bengal's *jatra* inspired Brajanath Sarma's theatre group, Achyut Lahkar's Nataraj theatre was inspired by the *Assam Kohinoor Opera Party*. Since its inception, mobile theatre has occupied a prominent place in Assamese public life. It did not remain confined to Pathshala or the region of lower Assam alone. With the improvement in transportation services and the building of better roads across the state, greater mobility was possible. Hence, these theatre groups started easily navigating between villages, towns, and cities within Assam. Therefore, although born in Pathshala, mobile theatre spread to Guwahati and the upper parts of Assam.

7.2.2 *Structure, Size, and Ownership*

Even though there are differences in how each mobile theatre group is formed and functions, similarities exist in their basic organisational structure. A mobile theatre group is owned by a producer and consists of at least 100–200 members. If one looks at the demographic composition of the groups, most members including producers come from lower strata of the society. They belong to lower castes and rural areas. The theatre group travels from one place to another within Assam—from villages to towns to cities as indicated by the word 'mobile.' When there is a performance, the whole troop travels to the host destination. The contingent moves with all the equipment, props, and costumes. Almost every group owns a truck or two, which is the primary vehicle of transportation from place to place.

The members comprise the producers, the actors, dancers, playwrights, musicians, singers, choreographers, technicians, sound artists, action artists, make-up artists, administrative and managerial people, and workers. Both men and women play these roles. The theatre party functions like a company, where the producer is the owner and the artists and workers are its employees. They are employed contractually for a particular season and may or may not be retained for the next season. All workers and artists have to sign legally binding contracts. They cannot go home for the duration of nine months that the theatre season is in operation, unless there is an emergency. The theatre parties hire many actors and other artists for a season, who may or may not be retained for the next season. Some actors are 'star attractions,' and theatre groups generally prefer keeping them for the next year as well. Mobile theatre groups are often family enterprises as the reign of the group is passed down from one generation to another.

There are divisions and gradings within theatre parties. There are class I troops like Kohinoor, Abahan, Brindaban, and Hengul; class II groups like Bordoisila and Bhagyadevi; and class III parties like Raj Tilak and Suraj. Rates of artists, performance fees, and audience turnover vary from class to class. There is an All Assam Mobile Theatre Association which has specific rules and regulations that govern the living conditions of artists.

7.2.3 Schedule and Season

The groups stage new plays each year—which are around 50–200 shows per year. The theatre season commences around July/August when the preparation of the plays begins. The actors set up provisional residences, travel, rehearse, and perform together. Men and women actors live together in closeness to each other while preparing for their performances. After almost two months of practice and groundwork, the theatre groups start performing around September/October; the scheduling coincides with important festivals in Assam like Durga Puja and Deepawali or Diwali. These are also the months which see moderately little rain.

This season stretches till April, that is, it lasts for at least eight to nine months, during which the theatre party is consistently on the move. The season ends on 12 April. It is a fixed date as one of Assam's most famous festivals Rongali Bihu, the Assamese New Year, commences on 13 April. As such, everyone wants to be with their families. Therefore, the starting date can vary for the different groups, but the closing date is the same.

Organisations and institutions like colleges, schools, and temples invite theatre groups and lend their field to the party for three days for their performance. The theatre companies can also be called by the village council and the municipal corporations of towns and cities (Ross 2017, 74). The theatres have a system of operation and function within it. There is a secretary in each theatre group who makes all the deals with the organising committees. They decide when and where the party will travel.

7.2.4 Organisational and Technical Aspects

The mobile theatre stage is built in a makeshift manner in the field of the school or college that invites the theatre group to perform. It is not constant as the place of performance keeps changing. It is therefore not a proscenium theatre or a permanent theatre hall. But there is a stage, and it is not an open-air performance unlike *jatra* or other forms of folk theatre. The group moves around with its trucks of equipment to make the stage, props, and costumes (Ross 2017, 66). Technologically, mobile theatres are different from other forms of theatre as the technology used by these groups is quite advanced. Overall, every mobile theatre group has twelve teams, and each team is dedicated to different departments. These twelve departments are advanced stage, running stage, acting, dance, music, light, settings, props, kitchen, management and administration, transportation, and costume.

7.2.5 The Significance of the Public

These are some of the basic features of mobile theatre, which have contributed to its popularity and sustenance. It is seen as a theatrical form that is made for the public. Achyut Lahkar, the founder of the modern form of mobile theatre and the producer of the Nataraj theatre group, had argued that it is '*theatre of the public, by the public and for the public*'. Ratan Lahkar—the ex-producer of the Kohinoor theatre group had said that '*all that we have achieved is because of the love of the audience, which has been loyal to us for decades*' (Ross 2017, 65). They highlight the importance of the public in the journey of mobile theatre.

But who constitutes this public? The public that watches mobile theatre is not uniform; it is not a singular entity. It is heterogeneous. Mobile theatre was never a product of and/or for urban middle-class people. It originated in a rural backdrop, and even today, a significant portion of its audience is rural. This permeability and non-conformity to the idea of a singular urban, male, and upper-class audience are those that make it a counter-public (Patgiri 2021). Mobile theatre of Assam cuts across region, language, class, and gender to exhibit characteristics of a counter-public which resists hegemonic ideas of art and performance. Mobile theatre is considered a crass medium of entertainment with no significance in the nation's political imagination by several drama critics. But people associated with mobile theatre see it as a voice of resistance that is non-elite and mass-centred.

One of the causes that explain mobile theatre's reach is its nature. It is mobile and moves from place to place. It goes to people on its own (Talukdar *in* Das 2018, 113). As many of the playwrights and producers say, '*mobile theatre is the only form of entertainment that goes to the people. It is important to bring culture and art to villages, and mobile theatre does that*'. Its popularity cuts across cities, towns, and villages. It is incredibly popular in suburban areas like Pathshala, Jamugurihat, Chatiya, Lakhimpur, Nalbari,

Rangiya, and Bongaigaon. These places do not have shopping malls, cinema halls, or multiplexes, but mobile theatre is readily available.

Thus, unlike other forms of entertainment, mobile theatre has managed to penetrate Assam's villages. Improvement in transportation facilities and the building of better roads have meant that it has become much more comfortable for theatre troops to go from one place to another, even to far-off regions. The portable character of mobile theatre has made possible its immense reach. Mobile theatre is not a 'concert piece' only for the modern, middle-class urban audiences. It makes theatre accessible also to the rural population. In both urban and rural areas, both men and women, almost in equal numbers, go to watch mobile theatre. Not just geographically, mobile theatre also bridges the gap among gender, class, caste, and ethnicity within the publics.

However, in the wake of the pandemic, people associated with mobile theatre felt that because of their popular nature, they were ignored. '*We are not taken seriously as an art form because of our nature. Be it the intellectuals or the government, nobody supported us. We were on our own*,' said one of the producers. This idea of being on one's own also shaped their responses to the challenges that mobile theatre faced during the pandemic. Resilience was the 'natural' response as there was no other option, as we will see in the next section.

7.3 Impact of the COVID-19 Pandemic: Challenges and Responses

7.3.1 Employment and Livelihood

Many people associated with mobile theatre make an association between employment and mobile theatre. The producers see it as a form of *jibika* (which means livelihood in English) and employment. '*Bhyrmoman soli ase kiyo nu manuh ok jibika diye, artist ok, local burok. (Mobile theatre is thriving because it provides livelihood to our artists and locals)*,' said one of the producers. The use of the word employment with theatre is paradoxical, as usually, being involved with theatre is seen as unstable and not 'real work.' But, as one organising committee member would argue, '*Axomor bhyrmoman xukiya hoi, local burok jibika dise. (Assam's mobile theatre is unique in many aspects. It is a significant form of providing work to locals).*' It has become a way of asserting Assamese local and cultural identity.

What is interesting to note is how mobile theatre and its accompanying skills are passed from one generation to the other. As a tradition that originated in the lower division of Assam, most of the theatre groups are based in that region. A majority of the artists, workers, and managerial people come from this division. For instance, a lot of young men who are involved in technical roles belong to the Goalpara district in the lower Assam division.

> *Goalparaor pora deka loar bur Barpeta ahisil kaam bisari. Settingsor xoru xura kaam xiki, gaot goi baaki buroku xikaise, utsah diye. Ei*

> *kaam burot iman porha xuna nalage seye koribo pare. (Young boys from Goalpara used to come to Barpeta looking for work. They learned these small technical works, and when they went back to their villages, they would teach others as well, motivating them. These jobs did not require much education and hence were easily available to such young boys)*, said a playwright.

Krishna Roy, the producer of the Abahan theatre group, for instance, initially worked in the technical department of Nataraj theatre under Achyut Lahkar in the 1960s. It was only much later that he became a producer. However, these skills have not always been generational or inherited. Initially, some of the young men from the Kamrup and Barpeta districts were sent to Mumbai to observe and understand how film sets are made, how studios are designed, and how sound and lighting are done. It was only later on that these skills and knowledge could be passed on from one generation to another.

Generating employment goes hand in hand with providing support to the local people. Mobile theatre is seen as a local art form that has sustained itself because of the involvement of local people. '*Nibonua xomosya iman barhi goise eitu xomoyot, kintu bhyrmomane kaam diye maunhok. (There is so much unemployment in Assam and mobile theatre supports locals by employing them in various kinds of work)*,' said one producer. The producers take a lot of pride in it, as they believe that it is one of the few local sectors that have managed to not only survive but also consistently do well. '*Pathshalar protitu poriyalor ejon holeu sdasya, kunubakhon nohoi kunubakhon aahbayak somitir soite jorito. (Every family in Pathshala has at least one member in the organizing committee)*,' said Ratan Lahkar, the ex-producer of the Kohinoor theatre group (Figo and Patgiri 2013, 98).

But during the pandemic, mobile theatre came to a complete halt. This has had a profound impact on the artists. The term artist here is important. As stated earlier, it does include not only the actors but all members of a theatre group. But the consequences of the pandemic have been uneven for the artists. While for actors there have been possibilities of engaging in other kinds of work, for technical and other workers, the impact has been particularly devastating.

Many artists started engaging in alternative forms of employment as their savings ran out. They started selling tea, vegetables, fruits, meat, fish, and eggs or engaged in daily wage work. Some others also migrated out of the state in search of better opportunities. Most of them are from rural as well as lower caste and class backgrounds with families to feed. Although they did not want to leave mobile theatre, they had no other choice. They were in a situation that can be characterised as 'no show, no pay.' Thus, one question that the producers dealt with is how the theatrical form survives in this situation. Unfortunately, there are no clear answers. The producers recognise that it would be difficult to bring the people who left back to mobile theatre. It is not easy for people to move from one job to another. Many have also migrated outside Assam, and as such, they might not want to come back. Thus, rural artists with marginal identities engaged in a theatrical form that caters to the public were pushed out of the space.

As stated earlier, the skills associated with mobile theatre are not taught in an institutional capacity. No theatre or drama school imparts the knowledge that is required to operate in a mobile theatre. As such, this knowledge is hereditary and passed on orally from one generation to another. Many also learn from watching rehearsals as there is a practicality attached to theatre. Therefore, the migration of artists from mobile theatre to other forms of employment is a severe threat to mobile theatre itself. Training new people and continuing this form of art is a very challenging task. There was a sense of theatrical displacement (Houlihan and Morris 2021).

The producers are also aware of the fact that several artists left the art form. But as many of them have argued, there is only so much that they can do. Mobile theatre units also face issues in procuring loans and financial help from banks as they are not seen as manufacturing units. This is a long-standing issue that is associated with the nature of mobile theatre itself. It is not a registered industry and this means that they cannot avail a lot of benefits that the state awards industries. In 2003, the All Assam Mobile Theatre Association told the government that mobile theatre should not be declared as an industry. This decision was taken to protect the autonomy of mobile theatre. But in light of the pandemic, it has been highly debated.

The producers, however, have argued that they did not have much of a choice. One cannot register mobile theatre as a society because each group is led by one producer. It is a sole proprietorship in operation but becoming a society requires more people to come together. Hence, it is not a feasible option. Nonetheless, in the face of the pandemic, there has been a general recognition that the role of the state has not been satisfactory in providing policy support. But a lot of people also said that they did not expect much from the government considering their past experiences. Since these artists have been without state safety nets even before the pandemic, they had no savings to fall back on. The crisis of marginality was acute.

Since the lock down was announced right before Rongali Bihu, a major festival in Assam, several shows were already in the pipeline. But they had to be cancelled. They were asked to stop their performances a month before their closing date. As such, producers suffered heavy losses and could not pay artists. The parties tried liaisoning with the government but they were not successful (Barman 2022).

7.3.2 State Responses to the Crisis

Many producers have argued that they were in constant dialogue with the state government. One proposal was to reduce the number of people in the audience and increase the number of shows. They have also stated that since mobile theatre happens on a makeshift stage, it is possible to maintain physical distance and space. While acknowledging the fact that none of these was going to be easy, they were willing to put forth their best foot forward to revive this unique theatrical tradition of Assam. They were looking at co-habitation with the virus in the context of the pandemic. There are, however, several practical and logistical concerns that impact these decisions. One is rising inflation. While the producers state that it is still possible to cut costs on props, costumes, and make-up, they cannot do that in two major aspects that define mobile theatre's sustenance—transportation and food. There was also a loss of several pieces of equipment, especially wooden and bamboo items that got damaged.

There was a crisis of public space, especially for performing arts and creative activities (Khofifah et al. 2022). An order was released by the Assam State Disaster Management Authority on 8 October 2021 (SDMA, Government of Assam 2021). It allowed theatres to operate at 50 per cent capacity with fully vaccinated attendees and organisers in response to continuous requests from mobile theatre troops. The order had several guidelines dictating how mobile theatres should operate. They were directed to get permission from the jurisdictional or sub-divisional district magistrate to conduct shows. Additionally, they were asked to fully vaccinate all members of the organising committee and the troops. Several other guidelines like closing the show on time, arranging thermal scanners and hand sanitisers, regular testing, and frequent announcements regarding the threat of the virus were to be followed.

One can see that the entire responsibility was on the theatre groups. For many producers, it was not possible to make such elaborate arrangements. One of them told me, '*I paid for the vaccination costs of many artists in my troop. But I cannot do it for the organizing committee members.*' Since the guidelines were so elaborate, not many schools or colleges wanted to take the burden of organising theatre. As such, even after the order was released, mobile theatre groups did not immediately return to work. It was a crisis that needed not just state directive but also support.

Some people had suggested collaborating with multinational corporations (MNCs) and generating money through sponsorships. However, the people associated with mobile theatre feel that this move will undermine its autonomy. Since the major attraction of mobile theatre is believed to be the commitment to its local roots, forming partnerships with international and/or national companies is seen as detrimental to local interests. For the producers of mobile theatre, generating employment has gone hand in hand with providing support to the local people. Mobile theatre is seen as a local art form that has sustained itself because of the involvement of local people. Therefore, this dependence on MNCs is not seen as desirable. However, some finances were generated through crowdfunding.

This is not the first time that mobile theatre has faced a crisis. When it was at its very nascent stage, Achyut Lahkar faced heavy losses and was unable to buy even groceries for his household. The Natraj theatre group was under such debt that all the artists left the group and it was almost dead. During that period, people from Pathshala helped him overcome this situation and stood by him. At one point in time, the budget of a theatre group was only 20,000–25,000 rupees but now the range is between 50 lakhs and 2 crores. This is the exponential growth that mobile theatre has seen. Similarly, rainy weather creates hurdles in performances of mobile theatre, as was seen in 2016. The state of Assam was plagued by massive floods in 2016, and mobile theatre had taken a hit that year. People faced many hardships to come to the venues, and it was also difficult for the theatre parties to build their makeshift stages. So the producers are optimistic that they will survive the COVID crisis as well.

But this is the version of the producers—the owners of the mobile theatre troops. Artists have their version of the story. Even before the pandemic, the nine-month contract period has been a bone of contention for artists. Because of temporary employment, they are deprived of a lot of social security measures that are availed by employees from other industries. The non-recognition of mobile theatre as an industry means that the employees are deprived of many benefits and provisions of labour laws.

7.3.3 Working Conditions

There is also job insecurity that the mobile theatre artists face, especially the supporting artists. Another cause of discontentment that the artists have is related to the leave policy that mobile theatre groups follow. It is difficult for them to get leave even in cases of emergency. Jitu Das, a technician who had worked with Hengul theatre committed suicide after he was not granted leave to see his ailing father who was on his deathbed. He lost his life because of the strict leave policy of mobile theatres.

Although mobile theatre is profitable and commercially viable, it is too top-heavy. There are hierarchies and divisions amongst the artists and workers like in all other industries, which are reflected in their wages, accommodation, lifestyle, and food. The top artists in mobile theatre earn 40–50 lakhs per annum. These top artists are mostly film and serial actors, who are called 'stars.' The stars prefer to work in mobile theatre over films and serials as they can earn much more money in the former. But earlier, this was not the case. There were no 'stars.' Everyone was an artist. The actors who worked in mobile theatre were all artists. There were divisions by age and number of years in theatre (seniority) and so there were senior and junior artists. Although there were no stars, differences in wages existed even then. The senior artists would earn 10,000 rupees per annum, and the junior artists would make around 3,000 rupees per year.

Today the difference in wages is much higher between the stars, artists, and the workers. '*The cooks get only 1000 rupees or so per month. They are given food and accommodation, so they accept it*,' said a playwright. '*The producer has to pay the stars. He spends most of his money there*,' he further adds. The worst affected are the girls who perform in the dance dramas. They earn less, around 1,000 rupees or so per month, and have to attend to the stars.

But the difference between the stars and others is not restricted to wages alone. It extends to their accommodation and food provisions as well. In earlier years, all the artists would stay together in the local school or college. '*Big actors like Mahananda Bora and Suren Mahanta would stay with all the junior artists in the school*,' stated a dramatist. Nowadays, the stars prefer to stay alone and need special accommodation and facilities. As already discussed, they are accommodated in houses of well-to-do families in the villages. During rehearsals, they are also hosted by the producer themselves in their houses. For instance, Abahan theatre has some of the biggest stars, including Prastuti Parashar (the highest-earning actor in mobile theatre for the past two years), and they are accommodated in the producer's house. Many stars do not even do their chores, and the girls who work in dance dramas are asked to wash their clothes and perform other daily activities.

The girls accept it because the living conditions in their homes are even worse. '*Here they get to eat and some money. At home, they have nothing. Their conditions are so bad that they cannot even afford two meals. This is much better for them*,' said a director. These girls, however, have no security. They might not be retained for the next season if the producer is not happy.

These issues of obtaining leave, pay differences, working and living conditions, etc. were exacerbated in the wake of the pandemic. Because of their preexisting precarity, supporting actors, technical artists, dancers, and other workers were the ones most affected by the pandemic. They had no savings and did not get paid when mobile theatre was shut down. Hence, most of them had to find alternative livelihood opportunities.

7.3.4 The Threat of Digitisation

Mobile theatre is also facing a major threat from digital modes of entertainment, particularly Over-the-Top (OTT) platforms. According to a report that was brought out by SBI Research (a division of MarketResearch.com), the OTT market is expected to reach Rs 11,944 crores by 2023, up from Rs 2,590 crores in 2018. The report published in August 2022 projected an annual growth of 36 per cent (Talukdar 2022). Thus, there is a stupendous rise in the consumption of OTT content. It is seen as a major threat to many other forms of entertainment like films and theatre.

But producers of mobile theatre believe that 'drama is drama.' It is a kind of live performance and has its unique attraction. It is human—there is no editing involved. They argue that digital content thus cannot present a threat to theatre and are optimistic that mobile theatre will survive this onslaught. In fact, mobile theatre is also a form of theatre that has adapted itself to the needs of the time. The primary purpose of mobile theatre has always been entertainment. It has survived because of the intimate connection that exists between the spectators and the performers. '*There is no point in shifting to digital performances as our USP is a connect with the rural audiences. It is live without any editing*,' said Nazrul Islam, the producer of the Bordoisila theatre group.

But one must also acknowledge that theatre parties have increasingly moved towards incorporating digital means in their live performances. The plays begin with title credits like it is done in films. It is displayed on a projector which is used over the stage to show the names of the actors, directors, writers, technicians, and the producer. This is a very recent development. Krishna Roy, the ex-producer of the Abahan theatre group, had told me during my fieldwork that it is their constant endeavour to create new things to keep the audience interested. '*Ami notun bostu, podhoti anar sesta kori thaku. Naam bur dekhai dile screentot shilpi aru kola kuxoli xokoleu olop gurutta pai. (We constantly try to introduce new things and techniques. If the names are displayed, the artists and the technicians also get a little recognition).*' It also helps the audience in getting to know who is acting in which play.

The trend of displaying title credits like films was started by the Abahan theatre group in 2015 and then later adapted by other theatre groups as well. Some groups nowadays also use pre-recorded music and songs in their plays. A projector is used to show flashbacks in certain scenes. Additionally, mobile theatre parties have effectively used YouTube to popularise their plays. The form and content of mobile theatre have undergone significant changes in recent years, and many plays contain song and dance sequences like films. Many parties 'release' videos of these songs on YouTube before the theatre season begins. This is similar to what movie production houses do with their music before the films are released. It is a tactic that mobile theatre parties use to create a buzz and sensation amongst the audience about their plays before the season starts officially. Many songs become extremely popular on YouTube, gathering millions of views. For example, *Oo maa* (O Mother) of the play *Mur Maar Suwali* (I Am My Mother's Daughter) by the Abahan theatre group is one of the most popular songs of the theatre season 2017–2018, which was made available on YouTube beforehand and has gathered at least 4.5 million views. Mobile theatre parties use YouTube also to release short promotional videos of their plays before the season begins officially. For instance, the Bordoisila theatre group released a video containing trailers of its three plays—*Deuta* (Father), *Grihalakshmi* (Housewife), and *Putola* (Doll)—that have been performed during 2018–2019.

Mobile theatre groups experiment with technology like lighting, sound, and music. For instance, the Kohinoor theatre group introduced 3D technology in their play *Breaking News* in 2016. Thus, there is a lot of engagement with both technology and digital media. Therefore, in my opinion, it would be premature to comment if mobile theatre will survive the digital onslaught as it is still an evolving story.

7.4 Conclusion

As has been discussed in this chapter, the impact of the pandemic on Assam's mobile theatre has been devastating. A form of activity that has been popular statewide for the generation of both employment and income was completely stalled in the pandemic. With the return to 'normalcy' in the post-COVID world, mobile theatre groups also resumed their operation in 2022. But not every group was able to restart. The newer ones struggled to cope with the effects of the pandemic, and the number of mobile theatre groups has declined.

Nonetheless, the theatre groups did see a ray of hope after the misery and crisis that they endured during the pandemic. Tapan Lahkar, the producer of the Kohinoor theatre group, said that the pandemic had left all of them miserable and hopeless. But now '*we see hope again*.' However, even then, not all groups have been able to make a comeback. The pandemic has altered how we envisage the world—the way we behave and engage with our local environments and cultural products. The private and public performing spaces have collided and the aesthetics of art have been forced to change for survival (Wadhwa and Kav 2021). Thus, only time can tell us how the public engages with mobile theatre in the post-pandemic situation. It is still an evolving story.

Note

1 The term artist in mobile theatre's context was first used by Achyut Lahkar, the founder of the Nataraj theatre group, the first modern mobile theatre group. He had thought that using the term artist would give a certain amount of respect and dignity to the people involved in its various aspects, be it performance or technical.

References

Assam State Disaster Management Authority, Government of Assam Order No. ASDMA. 28/2021/270. 2021, Government of Assam.

Awasthi, S. and Schechner, R. 1989. "Theatre of roots": Encounter with tradition. *The Drama Review* 33 (4): 48–69.

Banks, M. and O'Connor, J. 2021. "A plague upon your howling": Art and culture in the viral emergency. *Cultural Trends* 30 (1): 3–18.

Barman, P. 2022. The impact of Covid-19 pandemic on Bhrmyoman theatres of Assam. *Journal of Positive School Psychology* 6 (4): 6168–74.

Comunian, R. and Lauren, E. 2020. Creative and cultural work without filters: Covid-19 and exposed precarity in the creative economy. *Cultural Trends* 29 (2): 116–28.

Das, A. C. ed. 2018. *Axomiya Natya Porikroma*. Guwahati: Banalata.

Dinardi, C., Wortman, A. and Hernández, M. M. 2023. "It's been a roller coaster": Insights from performing artists on the Covid-19 pandemic and cultural policy. *Cultural Trends* 1–17. http://doi.org/10.1080/09548963.2023.2227865.

Figo, A. and Patgiri, P. 2013. *Bhyrmoman Theatreror Adhunik Khanikar Ratan Lahkaror Jiboni Grantha*. Pathshala: Writer's Forum.

Houlihan, B. and Morris, C. 2021. Introduction—performing in digital in the Covid-19 era. *Research in Drama Education: The Journal of Applied Theatre and Performance* 27 (2): 157–67.

Jones, S. 2022. Cracking up: The pandemic effect on visual artists' livelihoods. *Cultural Trends* 33 (1): 1–18.

Kalita, K. 2020. Covid-19 scare: Mobile theatre groups stare at uncertain future. *The Times of India*. Accessed 19 June 2024. https://timesofindia.indiatimes.com/city/guwahati/covid-19-scare-mobile-theatre-groups-stare-at-uncertain-future/articleshow/74650833.cms.

Khofifah, A., Werdiningtyas, R. and Kusumastuti, K. 2022. The changes in public spaces usages for performing arts sector after Covid-19 disruption in Surakarta, Indonesia. *IOP Conference Series: Earth and Environmental Science*. IOP Publishing Ltd.

Patgiri, J. 2021. Assam: Pathsala's great mobile theatre culture on last legs due to Covid-19. *EastMojo*. Accessed 19 June 2024. https://www.eastmojo.com/assam/2021/07/18/assam-pathsalas-great-mobile-theatre-culture-on-last-legs-due-to-covid-19/.

Patgiri, R. 2019. Mobile theatre of Assam: A socio-historical perspective. *Journal of North East India Studies* 9 (1): 29–51.

Patgiri, R. 2020. *Bhyrmoman Natak in Assam: A Study of Publics*, unpublished PhD dissertation, Jawaharlal Nehru University (JNU), New Delhi.

Ross, I. 2017. The mobile theatre movement in India: A success story in Assam. *New Theatre Quarterly* 33 (1): 65–77.

State Innovation and Transformation Aayog (SITA), Government of Assam. 2020. *Report on Economy of Assam: In the Backdrop of COVID-19 Pandemic*. Guwahati: State Innovation and Transformation Aayog (SITA), Government of Assam in Collaboration with Omeo Kumar Das Institute of Social Change and Development.

Talukdar, S. 2022. Is there any hope for revival of Assam's mobile theatre industry? *EastMojo*. Accessed 19 June 2024. https://www.eastmojo.com/assam/2022/09/03/is-there-any-hope-for-revival-of-assams-mobile-theatre-industry/.

Wadhwa, C. and Kav, S. 2021. Art at the edge: Performing arts in the pandemic. *Dhaara*. Accessed 19 June 2024. https://dhaaramagazine.in/2021/07/02/art-at-the-edge-performing-arts-in-the-pandemic/.

Part III

Frontline Workers, Caste Dynamics, and Labour Force

8 The Last of Frontline Workers

Casteism and Precarity among Sanitation and Waste Workers during COVID-19

Aparna Agarwal

8.1 Introduction

The outbreak of COVID-19 came as a major jolt to India's informal economy. The mass exodus of migrant workers to their home states was compared to the partition of India and Pakistan in 1947. The sudden announcement of lockdown by Prime Minister Narendra Modi left migrant workers in a vulnerable state, more out of the fear of joblessness and being away from home than the fear of COVID-19. However, given the state of panic and chaos throughout the country, essential services had to carry on. Doctors, police, medical staff, journalists, and cleaners (sanitation workers[1] and waste pickers), in the given order, were categorised as essential workers. Those who fell in this bracket of employment had no option but to go to work in person. Many of them received a standing ovation at their place of work and neighbourhood, and simultaneously, many were socially distanced and discriminated against. The story of these behaviours varies for different fields of work—medicine, police, and sanitation are quite different. While a large section of India's informal economy, such as domestic workers, construction workers, health care workers, and street vendors to name a few, experienced severe hardships and was driven to its extreme margins, cleaning workers endured pandemic-induced precarity, which was further compounded by exacerbated conditions of casteism, including enforced social and physical distancing. Following this, I examine the varying forms of discriminatory attitude and humiliation faced by cleaning work force and their changing forms during the pandemic and how a pandemic took the shape of 'casted' pandemic. At the beginning of the pandemic, the cleaning work force in many parts of the country was heralded as corona warrior, essential/frontline workers and there was a realisation that their work is pertinent in fighting against COVID-19. However, very soon, the discriminatory casteist attitude of middle-class residents and government officials came out in open—sometimes in a subtle manner and sometimes in a crude manner, as has been illustrated by Lee and Swaroop[2] and Rawat.[3] This then also informs us how the pandemic, which could have offered the potential for a more hopeful future, became a caste-driven crisis. Consequently, the lives of marginalised communities were further marginalised.

DOI: 10.4324/9781003591641-12

Historically, waste (mapping onto dirt), sanitary infrastructure, and epidemics were closely related. Historical scholarship on city-making in general and in Delhi (Prashad 2000[4]; Sharan 2014[5]; Chandavrakar 2009[6]) inform us that the growing fear of epidemics such as cholera and construing Indian cities as hotbeds of disease and unhygienic spaces led to segregation within the city. In the late 1880s, Bombay, Calcutta, and Delhi were the main focus of urbanisation. In order to maintain immaculate city centres and protect themselves from disease, it was necessary for the British to maintain clean and hygienic enclaved spaces within the city. These sanitised elite enclaves have been described by Guha as 'little islands of purity in the miasmatic landscape'.[7] One of the initial steps to control health, hygiene, and sanitation regulation in India was taken during the Crimean war.[8] As per the British authorities, approximately 10,000 British soldiers lost their lives during the war. Out of these 10,000 soldiers, 8,500 died as a result of diseases and unhygienic living conditions in India. Given this startling situation, the British authorities set up a Parliamentary Commission called 'The Sanitary Commission'. The Sanitary Report and Survey produced by The Sanitary Commission, analysed by Florence Nightingale, marked the beginning of the implementation of scientific ideas and modern sanitary practices in the country. One of her remarks regarding hygiene and sanitary conditions, as described in Waste of a Nation by Doron and Jeffrey,[9] was:

> The description given of the native town is astonishing. . . . So (far) as one judges from the evidence, the sanitary state of entire large cities is as bad as, if not worse than, was the state of the worst part of our worst towns before there was any sanitary knowledge in the modern world at all.
>
> (Sanitary State of the Army, p. 367. Cited in Doron & Jeffrey)

Given this highly negative description of 'contaminated' Indian cities, the British were able to carry out some sanitisation programmes in Indian cities, but they remained selective and focused mostly on the health and hygiene of British soldiers. It was only in 1882 when cholera and the bubonic plague (later 1890s) broke out in India that the British government accepted the germ theory and forced its techniques of modernisation on the Indian masses. With the spread of the plague in India, most of the British ships were barred from international trade. They were seen as carriers of germs and a potential cause of the spread of the plague to other European countries. The colonial government's vested economic interest forced them to impose sanitary practices on the Indians, which often meant intruding into Indian households. Arnold[10] and McFarlane[11] have argued that these processes of modernisation and sanitisation were mostly restricted to the British regiments and elite Indians. Slum colonies and working-class areas were left in deplorable conditions as they were beyond the budget of the British regime.[12] Their main priority was to treat the British bureaucrats and soldiers.

Furthermore, these unequal sanitary developments were followed by draconian measures, which meant enforcing strict quarantine rules, barging into private spaces of the natives, and demolishing their houses. The fear of such measures even led to widespread strikes and simultaneous arrests among sanitation workers (Mehtars) in Calcutta (now Kolkata). The word had spread among sanitation workers in Calcutta that authorities were forcibly taking workers to the hospitals and they should all follow the suit.[13]

We can see many such continuities and parallels in terms of unequal access to sanitary and waste management infrastructure in the postcolonial context, specifically in today's time of COVID-19–where in, though sanitation workers were initially applauded, later on they were forced to work in abysmal conditions. In fact these moments in history are often evoked to understand if the present-day pandemic will lead to major reforms in public health or sanitary infrastructure. For example, Swaroop and Lee in their essay on Caste and COVID-19 show how public health disasters in New York led to reforms in the working conditions of sanitation workers, including better wages and work hours, among many others. However, on the contrary, the present-day context and the conditions of sanitation and waste workers during the pandemic in Delhi, as sufficiently demonstrated in the subsequent sections, the process reveals an intensification of colonial and casteist attitudes towards sanitation and waste workers in the city.

Following the historical overview, we now turn to the contemporary scenario under the Swachh Bharat Abhiyan and its impact on sanitation workers during the pandemic. This will set the stage for examining the specific working conditions and systemic challenges faced by these workers in Delhi during COVID-19.

8.2 Swachh Bharat and Corona Warriors

Arguably, the moral and spiritual grounding of Swachh Bharat Abhiyan (SBA) considerably shaped the plight of sanitation and waste workers during COVID-19. Prime Minister Modi flagged off the SBA from Valmiki Basti, Mandir Marg, Delhi, on 2 October 2014. The Basti is historically significant because Gandhi stayed there for 214 days in 1946–47 and one of the main aims of his stay was to improve the living conditions of the Balmiki community, who form part of the sanitation workforce in the city. Even though Gandhi referred to sanitation work as spiritual work and that of cleaning the 'body of the society', yet he never really confronted the question of the caste order. Rather, he put the onus on the community of how an 'Ideal Bhangi' should be accepted in society. By moralising and eulogising the work done by 'Bhangis', he put the community on a pedestal but never questioned the fact of why only Bhangis should do this work. In fact, as Prashad[14] observes in his work, during Gandhi's initial visits to the Valmiki Basti, he referred to sanitation workers as 'Bhangi', and it was only later that he renamed them *Harijan*—children of god. Teltumbde[15] refers to this paternalistic attitude towards the caste system as 'muted casteism'. In his assertion of 'Mahatmahood' and by referring to cleaning work as a spiritual experience, Gandhi reinforced and legitimised the existing hierarchies of the caste system. His affirmation of the caste-based nature of sanitation work is conveniently appropriated by the present-day government under the SBA. Prime Minister Narendra Modi has time and again referred to cleaning work as a spiritual experience[16] and remarked that it is not simply work, but it is their (the Balmikis) duty to do this job for the larger good of society. In his famously authored book, Karamyog, Modi[17] states:

> I do not believe that they have been doing this job just to sustain their livelihood. Had this been so, they would not have continued with this type of job generation after generation. . . . At some point of time, somebody must have got the enlightenment that it is their (Valmikis') duty to work for the happiness of the entire society and the Gods; that they have to do this job bestowed upon them by Gods; and that this job of cleaning up should continue as an internal spiritual activity for centuries. This should have continued generation after generation. It is impossible to believe that their ancestors did not have the choice of adopting any other work or business.

It is very evident from this statement that by legitimising cleaning work in a paternalistic fashion—notwithstanding ongoing privatisation and informalisation of waste and sanitation work. Modi tried to deprive sanitation workers of their own identity and agency—in terms of how they (sanitation workers) view their own work. His applauding of cleaning work was followed by the theatrics of washing the feet of sanitation workers in Varanasi. Similarly, many have argued that Prime Minister Modi never used the 'C' word.[18] The 'C' word here refers to caste. Rather, the question of caste has been conveniently sanitised and muted. Gatade[19] observes how the Modi government conveniently ignored the agitation and effigy burning led by Dalits in Tamil Nadu in the wake of Modi's remark on cleaning work as a spiritual experience. Similarly, the government ignored the Safai Karamchari Aandolan's mobilisation against dry latrines. These observations demonstrate how the politics of symbolism around the SBA by eulogising the cleaning work and workers, albeit by invisibilising the question of caste, has further legitimised the discourse around the SBA and has complicated the socio-economic conditions of waste workers.

Such casteist Gandhian strategies were conveniently deployed even during the pandemic, wherein sanitation workers and waste workers were initially hailed as Corona warriors. Their work was revered as essential work to sustain clean, hygienic, and immaculate public spaces and mitigate any possible risk which could be caused by COVID-19. However, these labels and tags did not aid in significantly improving the socio-economic conditions of the cleaning workforce and the prevailing stigma associated with the work. On the contrary, as evidenced in the narratives below, the COVID-19 led conditions further pushed them on the brink of the precarious living and laid bare the already existing schisms of social hierarchy and physical distancing, further exacerbated by the practice of 'social' distancing. These conditions can be attributed to two main factors—the first is the caste-based morality of SBA, which furthers and legitimises the marginalisation of Dalit sanitation workers in the city, and the second is the ongoing informalisation and privatisation of sanitation and solid waste management services, respectively, in the city under the banner of SBA.[20] To briefly summarise the process: the ongoing informalisation among sanitation workers involves the contractualisation of work, where sanitation workers increasingly lack permanent jobs and must survive on a meagre salary of Rs. 13,000 (based on fieldwork conducted in 2019–2020), without any job security. Similarly, with respect to garbage collectors, the ongoing privatisation under a public–private partnership (PPP) has led to deplorable working conditions and marginalisation among informal waste pickers. Previously, informal waste pickers collected waste from middle-class households, local receptacles, and landfills. However, with the advent of PPP companies, their access to waste materials and, consequently, their daily earnings have significantly decreased. While these changes have been in progress for the last two decades, they have been further solidified and concretised under the banner of SBA.

8.3 Working Conditions of Sanitation Workers and Waste Workers During COVID-19

For many sanitation workers and waste workers, the pandemic highlighted, worsened, and reinforced the already existing work conditions and the caste hierarchies associated with the sanitation and waste workers. Given the nature of the pandemic, cleanliness and hygiene are so pertinent to its eradication that any kind of dirt, or disorder of waste, could prove to be disastrous. However, as it has historically been the case, the dirt had to be borne by the *Safai karamcharis* (sanitation workers) of Balmiki community, who have always been socially and physically ostracised and discriminated and in present-day times it is also borne by the informal waste pickers who are mostly from lower-caste communities, such as Schedule Caste (SC) and Hindu and Muslim OBCs.

The first day after the lockdown, it was a chaos for many sanitation workers and waste pickers, as many of them travel for 20–30 km on a daily basis to reach their workplace. Due to the lack of transportation facilities, many sat at home clueless. While it was announced that those who have to travel afar and have to cross borders, mostly from UP and Haryana, can stay at home. However, as it turned out a month later, their salaries where deducted for not reporting on those days. Similarly, early in the lockdown, many national dailies, such as *The Indian Express*, in Delhi reported that many sanitation workers (approximately 27,000) from the North Delhi

Municipal Corporation (NDMC) and mostly deployed on COVID-19 duty didn't receive their salaries for two months. Later I also confirmed the same based on a telephonic conversation. The pandemic had already made it difficult for many of them to afford their daily necessities, and the delay in their salaries made the situation still worse.[21] As soon as the delay in salaries became public knowledge, government authorities—both the Delhi government and North Delhi Municipal Corporation—started the blame game.

The East Delhi Municipality Corporation (EDMC), notoriously known for its corruption, followed the same path. As per the reportage in *The Times of India*, sanitation workers in East Delhi had not received their salary since December 2020, following which they resorted to strike on 16 January 2021. Usually, during these strikes, sanitation workers refuse to clean the streets and drains, and they often work in close cooperation with informal waste pickers and PPP-led waste management companies to stop them from collecting garbage. These strikes are further exacerbated by sanitation workers by throwing garbage on the streets. The strike held in the second week of January was no different, and its repercussions spread to areas across East Delhi. Concerned by the growing outrage among the middle-class residents of the city and the growing 'disorder' caused by the dumping of trash on the streets, the EDMC officials were forced to clear the dues of sanitation workers in the first week of February, following which the strike was called off. However, before the strike was called off, the EDMC filed a plea against sanitation workers for striking and for creating a nuisance for the public by stopping the PPP-led garbage removal trucks. As per the *Hindustan Times*' reportage, the EDMC's standing counsel, Manu Chaturvedi, argued in the court stating that the sanitation workers were protesting even though their salaries were cleared till December 2020.[22] The court bench comprising Justice Vipin Sanghi and Justice Rekha Palli came down heavily on the sanitation workers and said, '[E]veryone should realise that in a civilised society, such anarchy cannot prevail and it is essential to maintain rule of law and public order, so that all authorities including police can take measures to deal with the menace created by miscreants'. To this, they further added, '[W]e are observing that if the MCD employees have any grievance and resort to a legal strike that does not entitle them to take law into their own hands and create anarchy'. However, in order to protect the interest of the workers, the EDMC mayor gave the statement that 'the sanitation workers are like a family and that no legal action would be taken against any of them' (*Hindustan Times* 2020). Finally, the strike was called off when the EDMC cleared the prior dues. The statements made by the two judges and the EDMC mayor are emblematic of how these institutions look at the plight of sanitation workers. While the judges agreed that sanitation workers have the right to protest and resort to legal action, their active participation in the strike by resorting to dumping trash on the streets and waylaying garbage removal and threatening the drivers of private companies that continued to collect garbage was referred to as anarchy, and those who were involved in these actions were labelled 'miscreants'. It is ironic that depriving sanitation workers of two months' salary, that too during the pandemic—which could affect household expenditure, medical expenses, school/college of children, and delay in paying house rent—due to a lack of funds is accepted as the norm, whereas their active participation in a strike is referred to as anarchy. These instances were followed by furthermore lapses on part of the Municipal Corporation of Delhi (MCD), pushing them towards precarity and vulnerability.

It's a common site in the city to come across sanitation workers not wearing masks. They often prefer to cover their face with a handkerchief or their *Dupattas* (scarf). Once I was standing in the office of Assistant Sanitary Inspector (ASI) in North Delhi Municipal Corporation[23] ward, and a *safai karamchari* walked in without a mask. Looking at me, feeling conscious of his image, the ASI shouted at the karamchari 'where is your mask?' The worker shouted back, 'when you don't give us any masks and sanitisers, what do you expect us to do in this meagre salary!' Although, initially workers were given masks, they were unsure if masks could be used repeatedly, given that they are exposed to dust and waste daily. Few others complained that they were provided with masks but not gloves and sanitisers. Many workers expressed the need for sanitisers given the nature of their work. Instead, they were provided with fluorescent jackets so that they could be identified as 'essential' workers and not harassed by the police.[24]

These indifferent and careless treatments meted out by sanitation workers were further accentuated by practices of untouchability carried out at the quotidian level, adding insult to the injury. As I talked to one of the sanitation workers, A1, in Delhi's Ram Manohar Lohia Hospital, who has been working there for 15 years as a contractual labour with Sulabh International (where almost 700 *safai karamcharis* were working in different wards of the hospital), he told me that the everyday casteism is so normalised that the sanitation workers have stopped bothering about it. If we think about all this, how will we work. He said, 'madam, jaatiwad toh hai hi, ye toh humane sochna hi band kar diya hai. Aagar ye sab sochenge toh kaam kaise karenge'. The instances of sisters discriminating against them, not sharing their water and food with the sanitation workers is a very common practice. What becomes exceptional, yet normalised, is how lives of *safai karamcharis* are rendered secondary to everyone else working in the hospital. While doctors and nurses work closely with COVID-19-affected patients, it is the sanitation workers who ultimately get exposed to the urine and faeces of COVID-19 patients and PPE kits of doctors and nurses. Yet they hold the most precarious position in the frontline workforce. One of the karamchari aggressively remarked, '[H]ospital does not bother whether we live or die, at least 100 karamcharis have contracted COVID-19, but hospital didn't bother about our health and didn't consider giving us paid leaves. We are the ones who deal with the bodies, whether be it their blood, urine—we are the ones cleaning it'.

In the beginning of the COVID-19 pandemic, when there were not enough PPE kits, everyone was operating in the corona ward without proper safety equipment; if any doctor or nurse contracted COVID-19 they were quarantined in The LaLiT hotel (a five star hotel in New Delhi), or even if they did duty of straight 15 days, they were asked to stay in The LaLiT, whereas in the case of *safai karamcharis*, they had no option but to go back to their houses and many a times without even any proper transport facilities. To make the situation worse, contract-based *safai karamcharis* do not usually have any health insurance. However, back in 2020, Sulabh International started employee state insurance scheme (ESI) facilities for the *karamcharis*, which was also funded by karamcharis themselves. Prior to the ESI facility, their salary was Rs 15,000/month, but with ESI facilities and a deduction of Rs 2000, they received only Rs 13,000.

Similarly, as explained by the then chairman of Safaikaramchari Ayog (in August 2020) Sanjay Gehlot, many sanitation workers who died because of Corona while being on duty were not given compensation by the municipal corporations. Many a times, authorities tried to declare that the victims died of some other causes instead of corona in order to not provide compensation. Here, the *safai karamcharis* become a bate in the hands of central and state governments, which conveniently shifted their burden on to each other.[25] Delhi government often claimed, the moment they get the report from the concerned MCD commissioner about the death of a *karamchari*, they will release the money. However, as per the Delhi government (back in July-August-September 2020), they did not receive the death reports from the MCD commissioner, as claimed by *karamcharis*. Furthermore, on many occasions, sanitation workers had to collect money from their community members and activists for the treatment of COVID-19. They did not receive any substantial financial aid from the municipal corporations.

To make the matter worse, in the middle of the pandemic, the central government started the process of contractualisation of waste workers job with full force wherein no worker would have a permanent job and will be based on contract held by private companies. These processes have already been in the pipeline for many years, where the MCD has been pushing in private companies to take over the sanitation work.[26] The job of sanitation workers is divided into three categories—permanent, temporary, and casual workers. Permanent workers, as the name suggests, have a permanent job, are relieved from the services at the age of retirement, and get regular increments in their salary. Temporary workers, on the other hand, perform the same task but can be fired at any time and are not eligible for regular salary increments. Most of them have been getting Rs 13,000 per month for many years and are not eligible for any kind of promotion at the job. Moreover, casual workers are recruited based on demand, that is, when a permanent worker is on leave, and they are reimbursed for their work accordingly. Such conditions forced municipal *karamcharis* to protest in the middle of the pandemic.

The conditions of informal waste pickers were far worse than *safai karamcharis* and PPP-led garbage collectors during the pandemic. Unlike the latter two, the informal waste pickers are self-employed and do not have a steady flow of income. They rely on the availability of scrap materials, which they sell to the scrap dealers post-collection and earn money. Palpably, during the pandemic, the possibilities of picking up scraps became bleak for various reasons. The first reason was a considerable reduction in the availability of office waste and hotel-industry waste because of the lockdown. The second reason was that the stringent policing during the lockdown made it difficult for the waste pickers to access the middle-class colonies, local receptacles, and even landfills for that matter. It took some time for waste pickers to find their ways for picking up waste. Initially, as narrated by one of the waste pickers in my colony, they could not access the middle-class colonies because of heavy police deployment and had to dodge the police to reach their place of work. Furthermore, with the complete breakdown of supply-chain system, it was challenging to sell the *maal* (scrap materials). The waste pickers could not find any buyers for their *maal* and this was understandably followed by drastic fall in the prices of those materials. Many of them had collected *maal* before the pandemic and were looking for the right time to sell. But as soon as the pandemic hit, they were unable to sell even the previously collected maal.

Yet, the waste pickers continued to put their lives in danger and went on picking up waste. Waste picking in itself is quite a hazardous task and it was further accentuated during the pandemic. In order to increase the volume of the scrap materials, many waste pickers picked up COVID-19-related waste, such as personal protective equipment (PPE) suits, gloves, and face shields, and sold them to scrap dealers. One of my informants told me, '[A]nyway we deal with all kinds of waste on a daily basis. There is certainly an increase in medical waste, but prior to COVID-19 also, we saw half-dead animals, syringe and blood around the landfill. We are not surprised and bothered by the current situation. The moment we jump into the waste work, we leave our destiny to god. That is all we have'. COVID-19 has not stopped them limiting their already existing dangerous work conditions but has further pushed into one.

Maidul, a petty scrap dealer, who was one of my key informants, was forced to climb up the landfill during the lockdown due to a lack of earning. As a scrap dealer, Maidul had stopped picking-up waste for a few years and would only engage in buying and selling off waste. In one of our conversations he said, 'ab hum khaali babuaana kaam karte hain', meaning now he does not do physically laborious work. However, perilous economic conditions of COVID-19 pushed him to rummage for waste in and around the landfill, bringing him down to the ranks of waste pickers.

8.4 Everyday Casteism of Middle Class, COVID-19, and Waste Workers

After Prime Minister Narendra Modi declared the lockdown, there was utter chaos in the middle-class colonies the next day. While most of the migrant workers across the country were uncertain about their future and travelled back to their home states, the sanitation workers and many waste pickers stayed back.[27] Noticeably, sanitation and waste collection services were disrupted across the city. I recollect my own experience of 24 March, when everybody in my residential area was clueless about the waste collection and cleaning services. The informal garbage collectors were nowhere to be seen. The *safai karamcharis,* who usually come around 8 a.m., came around 11 a.m. By that time, an exasperated *Baniya* (a dominant trading caste) neighbour shouted, '[T]hese Bhangis just need a chance to skip their work. Now that we are in a lockdown, are we going to live with this dirt around us?' Soon, public–private partnership (PPP)-based waste-management agency came in (a PP partnership between a private company and the NDMC. On normal days, they compete over access to waste with informal garbage collectors, but on the morning of 24 March, all the burden of waste collection fell on their shoulders. Everyone wanted to dump their trash in the privately owned truck. Very soon, the truck outran its capacity, but the residents kept on dumping their trash, which eventually spilt out on the roads. This then led to another crisis—who would clean the roads in the absence of sanitation workers? Residents urged the PPP-led waste collectors to clean the streets, but when they refused, the residents were forced to pick up the scattered trash and dump it in the truck the next day. The next day residents complained to the municipal officers about the 'non-abiding' behaviour of the PPP-led waste collectors and from the next day NDMC officials made sure that the waste collection services in the area are not interrupted and that residents do not have to 'forcefully' dump their trash in the truck.

Very soon (in a week's time), when the informal waste pickers managed to make their way to the middle-colonies for garbage collection, they were meted out with unusual waste-collection practices. Typically, when handing over garbage dustbins, the middle-class colony residents often expect the informal garbage collectors to collect their garbage bins from their household, which many-a-times include climbing up the multi-storey buildings and cleaning of the stairs post-collection.[28] Furthermore, the waste pickers are often expected to clean the dustbins and then give it back to the residents. Although reluctant to clean the dustbins, the collectors do not have any option but to comply as otherwise the middle-class colonies' residents end up labelling them as rowdy and callous. Interestingly (and expectedly), the COVID-19 pandemic put an end to this practice of garbage collectors entering middle-class households. Seen as potential carriers of the virus, many households prohibited the entry of garbage collectors into their neighbourhoods. Instead, they would keep their dustbins outside their houses and wait for garbage collectors to come and collect the waste. Additionally, many households who would not usually cover their dustbins with a dustbin bag started covering their dustbins with a dustbin bag so that garbage collectors could not 'touch' their dustbins. Moreover, when household members contracted the virus, they would inform neither their neighbours nor their garbage collectors so as to ensure uninterrupted service of garbage collection and other everyday activities. Such questionable practices undoubtedly leave a negative impression on garbage collectors who put their lives at risk every day in order to serve middle-class residents. Thus, these inconsistencies about the entry of garbage collectors in the household domain are reflective of their prejudice based on their upper-caste privilege and paranoia regarding waste workers and how they choose to patronise them in order to maintain social boundaries and their own 'health' and 'safety', and show how the casteist practices of 'touch' and maintaining boundaries are conveniently reversed to adapt to the suitability of upper-caste concerns.

8.5 Conclusion

Given these narratives and explanations, I argue, the pandemic—which could have been a moment to understand the layered processes of waste management and sanitation services in Delhi and its adverse consequence—has been further exploited to reinforce and exacerbate the already existing social hierarchies and inequalities. Early into the pandemic it was envisaged that the beginning of COVID-19 might serve as a turning point in improving the state of public health and sanitary services in the country. Following the lessons from the history, as evidenced by Chandavarkar,[29] it was hoped that the central or state government might invest in public infrastructure facilities[30] and improve the conditions of essential workers. However, much to everyone's dismay, the socio-economic conditions of sanitation workers and waste workers severely deteriorated. Today, with the increasing privatisation of waste management services in Delhi, the deteriorating working conditions of waste workers are further worsened by the dominance of brahminical attitude of middle-class and the state-led bodies. The start of COVID-19 laid bare not only the vulnerable and precarious work conditions but also the varied forms of discrimination faced by 'essential workers' placed lowest in the hierarchy of work. These narratives reveal the stigma associated with waste work and also how it operates differently at multiple levels—sanitation workers, PPP-led workers, and informal waste workers. The distinction of public/private and informality have shaped the terms and conditions of work, yet what ties them together is the nature of waste work and the stigma associated with it.

While there is a need for major restructuring of the sanitary infrastructure in Delhi, much of the restructuring in the city entails technological 'advancement', furthering the comforts of upper-caste and class residents of the city. Such changes in the infrastructure are highlighted by the casteist attitude of government officials and residents of the city, who perpetuate discriminatory and inequitable behaviour towards the sanitary and waste work force in the city.[31] Moreover, even though early into the pandemic sanitation workers and waste workers were greeted with garlands and there was an apparent new found respect for them in the eyes of city's residents, which even workers were cognizant of, much of it soon faded as COVID-19 took hazardous and prolonged form. The respect was conveniently replaced by everyday casteism, self-preserving safety measures by middle-class residents, such as not informing garbage collectors if they contracted COVID-19, and informalisation of the sanitation workforce, as evidenced in the narratives above.

Notes

1 Here sanitation workers are defined in terms of sweepers (*safai karamcharis*) and waste workers are understood in terms of informal waste pickers who frequently make their way to middle-colonies and climb up the landfills to pick up discarded materials, followed by public–private partnership-led garbage collectors who provide household garbage collection services. PPP-led garbage collectors are hired by the companies on a contractual basis.

2 Kanthi Swaroop, and Joel Lee, Caste and Covid-19: Notes on sanitation in a pandemic, *Economic & Political Weekly* 56 (13) (2021): 35–42.

3 Vidya, Bhushan Rawat, Corona, caste and the lives of sanitation workers, *Countercurrents.org*, 10 July 2020. Accessed 10 February 2022. https://countercurrents.org/2020/07/corona-caste-discrimination-and-the-lives-of-sanitation-workers/.

4 Vijay Prasad, *Untouchable Freedom*, New Delhi: Oxford University Press, 2000.

5 Rajnarayan Chandavarkar, *History, Culture and the Indian City*, Cambridge: Cambridge University Press, 2009.

6 Rajnarayan Chandavarkar, *History, Culture and the Indian City*, Cambridge: Cambridge University Press, 2009.

7 Sumit Guha, Nutrition, sanitation, hygiene, and the likelihood of death: The British army in India c. 1870–1920, *Population Studies*, 47 (3) (1993): 385–401, 389.

8 Veena Talwar Oldenburg, *The Making of colonial Lucknow, 1856–1877*, Princeton, NJ: Princeton University Press, 1984.

9 Assa Doron, and Robin Jeffrey, *Waste of a Nation: Garbage and Growth in India*, Cambridge, MA and London: Harvard University Press, 2018: 18.

10 David Arnold, Pollution, toxicity and public health in metropolitan India, 1850–1939, *Journal of Historical Geography* 42 (2013): 124–33.

11 Colin Mcfarlane, Governing the contaminated city: Infrastructure and sanitation in colonial and post-colonial Bombay: Governing the contaminated city, *International Journal of Urban and Regional Research* 32 (2) (2008): 415–35.

12 Awdhendra Sharan, *In the City, Out of Place: Nuisance, Pollution, and Dwelling in Delhi, C. 1850–2000*, New Delhi: Oxford University Press, 2014.

13 Agarwal Prerna, The government will come to its senses, *The India Forum*, 30 April 2022. www.theindiaforum.in/authors/prerna-agarwal.

14 Vijay Prasad, *Untouchable Freedom*, New Delhi: Oxford University Press, 2000.

15 Anand Teltumbde, No Swachh Bharat without annihilation of caste, *Economic and Political Weekly* 49 (45) (2014): 11–12.

16 Ravichandran Bathran, The many omissions of a concept: Discrimination amongst scheduled castes, *Economic & Political Weekly* 47 (5) (2016): 30–35.

17 Narendra Modi, *Karamyog*, Government of Gujarat, 2007: 48.

18 Anand Teltumbde, No Swachh Bharat without annihilation of caste, *Economic and Political Weekly* 49 (45) (2014): 11–12.

19 Subhash Gatade, Silencing caste, sanitising oppression: Understanding Swachh Bharat Abhiyan, *Economic and Political Weekly* 50 (44) (2015): 29–35.

20 For a detailed discussion, see Olivia Calleja's (2021) work on public–private partnership of SWM services and informalisation of sanitation work in Delhi. Olivia

Calleja, 'Contingent resistance: The politics of waste commons in neoliberal Delhi, *Contributions to Indian Sociology* 55 (3) (2021): 416–37.

21 Abhinav, Rajput, Delhi: North body teachers, sanitation staff say not paid for 2 months, *The Indian Express*, 26 April 2020. https://indianexpress.com/article/cities/delhi/north-body-teachers-sanitation-staff-say-not-paid-for-2-months-6374803/.

22 Richa, Banka, Anarchy can't be tolerated: Delhi High Court on sanitation workers' strike, *Hindustan Times*, 6 February 2020. Anarchy can't be tolerated': Delhi High Court on sanitation workers' strike|Latest News Delhi—Hindustan Times

23 Around the time when the fieldwork was conducted, that is, from July 2019 to July 2021, the municipal corporation of Delhi was divided into three parts—North, South, and East. However, in March 2022, the three municipal corporations were integrated again.

24 Aparna Agarwal, The murky underbelly of sanitation during the pandemic, *The Wire*, 6 April 2020. https://thewire.in/rights/lockdown-delhi-ragpickers-sanitation-workers.

25 Arunabh Saikia, These frontline workers died of Covid-19. Their families are now struggling to get insurance money, *The Scroll*, 29 June 2020. https://scroll.in/article/968700/these-frontline-workers-died-of-covid-19-their-families-are-now-struggling-to-get-insurance-money.

26 N. A., No safai sainik will lose job: SDMC, *The Times of India*, 25 October 2020. https://timesofindia.indiatimes.com/city/delhi/no-safai-sainik-will-lose-job-sdmc/articleshow/78853412.cms.

27 Since sanitation job is based on hereditary rights, most of the sanitation workers in Delhi are from Delhi. Even though the workers are recruited via formal procedures, they usually inherit the job from their parents. Hence, with the imposition of the lockdown, the sanitation workers did not have to travel back to their home states. Whereas in case of informal waste pickers, most of them are migrant workers, they usually hail from West Bengal, UP, and Bihar, and many of them were forced to travel back to their home state in search for security and stability.

28 Collection of garbage sometimes leads to dirtying of stairs and informal waste pickers are expected to clean the stairs post-collection.

29 Rajnarayan Chandavarkar, *History, Culture and the Indian City*, Cambridge: Cambridge University Press, 2009.

30 Kanthi Swaroop, and Joel Lee, Caste and Covid-19: Notes on sanitation in a pandemic, *Economic & Political Weekly* 56 (13) (2021): 35–42.

31 Dana Kornberg, Garbage as fuel: Pursuing incineration to counter stigma in post-colonial urban India, *Local Environment* 24 (1) (2019): 1–17. https://doi.org/10.1080/13549839.2018.1545752.

9 COVID and Other Crises

Brick Kiln Workers and the Dismal Work Season of 2019–2020

Pratik Mishra

9.1 Introduction

The tragedy of COVID-19 and India's nationwide lockdown in March 2020 brought forth a reckoning of the scale of labour that is used up and discarded in the making of our cities. At a time when staying home was beseeched as a national duty, thousands upon thousands of migrant workers seemed to blatantly defy social distancing norms, crowding at bus stations, walking on highways and train tracks, seeking to return home. Around that time, I called a brick kiln worker, someone I had interviewed for my doctoral research and whose phone number I had, fearing he and his family may have become part of this mass exodus, leaving the brick kiln in northern India (in Khanda village of Sonipat District) for their village in far-off Bihar in the east of India. Reassuringly, they had not left the kiln, and migrant workers in nearby brick kilns of Khanda village were also mostly staying put. The spatiality of brick kilns in Khanda (true for brick kilns in general), being located as relatively isolated enclaves outside village or town residential centres, as well as their internal layout where work (and life) for most kiln workers is carried out in a decentralized manner, made brick kilns naturally conducive for social distancing. The brick kilns in Khanda are also clustered together densely with thousands of workers, and so were more easily visible for the local administration as a population centre than urban workers in scattered settlements. For the initial phase of lockdown, the local administration instructed brick kiln owners to manage basic provisions of food and supplies for kiln workers averting the crisis of food and rent that drove workers out of cities. Many brick moulding worker families continued to mould bricks on the workspaces adjacent to their homes, even in the midst of the strict lockdown. It would seem then at a glance that brick kiln workers were not experiencing the wholesale disruption to life and livelihood from the lockdown, that was afflicting migrant workers everywhere else. Indeed, the brick kilns of Khanda manifested as places of safe refuge during the lockdown for the sons and relatives of middle-aged brick kiln workers who were working in neighbouring areas of Delhi-NCR[1] in different urban and factory jobs.[2]

DOI: 10.4324/9781003591641-13

Staying at the kilns during the lockdown, however, was not much different from being stuck in the kilns. Most kilns stopped production and many workers had no income, sustaining themselves on basic food supplies from brick kiln owners. It is through considering the structural conditions of debt and precarity within the brick kiln labour regime that one can grasp the disruption and disturbance that the pandemic brought to kiln workers' livelihoods.

This chapter describes the unfolding of the COVID-19 pandemic within the brick kilns of Khanda and the lifeworlds of its inhabitants. It highlights the socioeconomic crisis of the COVID lockdown paying attention to how the lockdown led to several other crises for brick kiln workers. In doing so, the chapter seeks to decentre COVID-19 as an 'exceptional crisis' within the experiential frame of brick kiln workers, rather than understanding the pandemic in relation and continuous to the structural crises of work and life within the brick kiln. The pandemic however also functioned as a 'crisis of exception' with regard to the socio-cultural context of strangeness as fear, rumours, and indifference to the virus emerged in the kilns. This chapter further engages with this specific 'strange' nature of lockdown restrictions, delineating it as a crisis of exception but not as an exceptional crisis.

The chapter follows the period of disruption imposed within brick kiln workers' lives in Khanda for the entire eight-month-long brick-making work season from October 2019 to June 2020. The COVID lockdown beginning in March 2020 impacted workers who had already witnessed the paralysis of all work for over three months at the beginning of the work season (October to January). This was caused by the 'unexpectedly stringent' enforcement of the ban on brick kiln firing because of air pollution restrictions across Delhi-NCR. Kiln owners having to halt work were able to transfer the majority of the adverse economic impact of this ban onto wageless workers pushing them into an acute crisis of income and social reproduction.

How workers would later recount to me the economic burden of the COVID lockdown of 2020 was through a narrative of the general crisis of the 2019–2020 work season, merging the precarity imposed through both the incidents (as well as spates of irregular rainfall in February of 2020 that disrupted work). In writing this chapter, I mirror workers' accounts and present the livelihood shock of the pandemic in 'continuous' terms while not downplaying kiln workers' experiences of fear and the anxiety of epidemic during the COVID-19 lockdown period. For brick kiln workers who were simultaneously connected to the global discourse on COVID-19 through the internet and hearsay as well as disconnected through isolation and impediments of illiteracy, the risk of the COVID virus was interpreted through cultural matrices of epidemic-lore, superstition, rumours, and science. [This resonates with the book's premise that the COVID-19 crisis, as experienced by marginal migrant workers in India, is articulated through grief and pain much more than strangeness.]

Such an analytical frame has political implications. While scholars have emphasized the possibility for crises to serve as generative moments that open up internal contradictions otherwise submerged in the everyday,[3] the lockdown's continuity with precarious life in the kiln diminishes the possibility for structural critique to develop within such moments. For capitalist kiln owners and managers, the handling of the COVID-19 crisis continued on protocols executed in the previous air pollution ban, namely a drastic reduction in salaries for salaried workers, along with wagelessness and meagre rationing as debt for worker-households through local shops for (debt-bonded) piece-rate workers. The lockdown prepared no significant grounds for challenging the status quo of the labour regime that is structurally exploitative. At a broader scale, this was also reflected in how several Indian states like Madhya Pradesh and Uttar Pradesh responded to the pandemic by suspending protective labour laws and diminishing workers' rights in favour of capital, for instance, by increasing the permitted working hours from eight to twelve hours a day, without paying overtime.[4]

The public health concerns of COVID-19 were negotiated within a context where kiln workers remain unable to afford or access formal or qualified healthcare, save for a few life occasions. It is this exclusion that makes it unlikely that a scientific discourse on the virus will filter through to replace traditional modalities of understanding the disease and contagion. That brick kilns workers in Khanda were quite unaffected by COVID incidence in 2020 likely owes more to the natural conditions of habitation in the kilns and general public health measures than to informed action and vigilance by workers.

9.2 Methodology

This chapter largely draws from my doctoral fieldwork of over 11 months with brick kiln workers in Khanda as well as subsequently several post-PhD fieldwork visits since 2022 when I have also been engaged in a filmmaking project on brick kiln workers. Given that the chapter draws largely on the work season of 2019–2020, my fieldwork coincided with this season between September and December 2019 when I witnessed the crisis occasioned upon kiln workers from the air pollution-linked ban on brick kiln firing. The data on the effects of the COVID-19 lockdown was collected through telephonic interviews with known brick kiln workers and local villagers, as well as from subsequent fieldwork from April 2022. While my original doctoral research consisted of several interviews with 67 brick kiln workers as unique respondents, 39 of whom were brick moulders, a much smaller subset of 7 known workers were respondents for telephonic interviews on tracing COVID-19 lockdown impacts, as well as around 10 workers in post-PhD fieldwork. Aside from the workers, I also interviewed four villagers, and especially Dharmveer Singh, who is local to Khanda village and was previously my Research Assistant, was instrumental in providing me regular updates on broader village and brick kiln happenings during COVID. He did not visit any kilns but since the village's economy is tightly bound up with the kilns, he was a valuable source of general information on the happenings within the brick kiln-village complex (I compensated him for this help). The phone calls with brick kiln workers were not recorded; however, the purpose of the call to collect data was conveyed to informants and notes were taken by hand. Workers' names have been pseudonymized throughout the chapter.

Among several occupations within the brick kiln, my research was overwhelmingly focused on the brick moulders or *pathers* who often migrate with their families and live in the brick kilns for the full brick season. Moulders also make up the majority of workers (more than 70%) of any brick kiln in this area. I deal here exclusively with the politics of work surrounding the moulding occupation. The words brick moulder and brick kiln worker or brick worker are used interchangeably throughout this report.

Temporally, this chapter focuses on the 2019–2020 period which coincided with the first phase of COVID lockdowns between 24 March and 1 July 2020. While the second wave of the COVID-19 outbreak between March and May 2021 was more devastating in terms of mortality, the impact upon migrant brick kiln workers was pronounced during the first phase of the COVID lockdown in 2020. The first phase was much more marked as a period of economic shock and reverse migration from cities and other migrant destinations for informal workers. The workers I had been in touch with had all decided not to migrate to brick kilns of North India in September 2020 for the 2020–2021 work season, instead preferred to work in brick kilns or other occupations within their native regions of Bihar or Chhattisgarh. There weren't many brick kiln workers in Khanda for the 2020–2021 season and it was a weak year of brick production. Though there were some deaths among Khanda villagers from COVID-19 during the second wave of the pandemic, I did not hear of any brick kiln worker who had died from COVID-19 in Khanda during this period.

In the following section, I contextualize the research with a description of the field site of Khanda as well as a brief description of the labour regime within its brick kiln cluster. The orientation within this chapter as well as my broader research has been to approach the brick kilns as primarily a space of social reproduction for migrant brick kiln workers living there and secondarily as the productive space of the factory. The subsequent section discusses the work season of 2019–2020 as a temporal frame for establishing the continuity of precarious work and life throughout, including the COVID-19 lockdown, the air-pollution-linked stoppage of work, as well as the regular relations of brick kiln work in 'more normal' periods. The aspects of the labour regime along which continuity is traced are firstly, the imposition of unproductive idle time for kiln workers,[5] secondly, the provisioning of kiln workers with bare supplies instead of income during crises, and finally, the deduction of debt and allowances from kiln workers' earnings due to which workers often have to return empty-handed even after months of living and working at the brick kiln. Alongside the continuity of the experience of precarity, I also highlight the discontinuities of the pandemic lockdown to other periods, especially within the inability to secure basic resources with the shutdown of the market economy around the kilns. While reproductive life in the kilns is defined by material scarcity, the lockdown worsened this condition as workers were unable to access various market and resource spaces. In the final empirical section, the chapter describes the way by which kiln workers negotiated the public health understanding of the virus.

9.3 Contextualizing the Brick Kiln Cluster of Khanda

Khanda village, where I conducted my doctoral fieldwork research, is in Sonipat district, which is in the neighbourhood of Delhi and is part of the Delhi-NCR urban agglomeration. While Khanda has a population of about 12,000 local villagers who live within its residential area, the farmlands around Khanda are the site for over 60 brick kilns that together employ and house over 30,000 migrant workers for the eight-month long brick season, many workers migrating and living with their families. Khanda is a key village within the Kharkhoda brick kiln cluster, which is the second-largest cluster supplying bricks to Delhi-NCR.

Most brick kiln moulders in Khanda are migrants from the states of Bihar in eastern India or Chhattisgarh in central India. Migration and work in brick kilns is structured through the system of debt bondage, an unfree labour relation that has been prohibited under the Bonded Labour System (Abolition) Act, 1976, but continues ubiquitously as the norm for the industry. Recruitment of most workers including brick kiln moulders to the kilns is carried out through informal intermediaries called labour contractors or *jamadar* who offer workers in their native village, from their own funds or through funds from the kiln owner, a lump sum wage advance called *peshgi* as debt before migration to the kilns roughly around October. The wages for brick kiln moulders are on a piece-rate basis, as a fixed amount per 1,000 bricks moulded. The full wages are however kept in abeyance till the end of the season and only a stipend or allowance called *kharcha* is given to kiln-bound workers every fortnight for the purchase of basic supplies including alcohol. The final *nikas* or take-home wage is disbursed at the end of the brick season in June and calculated by deducting the *peshgi* and all the *kharchas* of the brick season from the full wages for all bricks moulded. The *nikas* can be, and often is, marginally positive, zero or negative if there are not enough bricks produced for various reasons (very often this happens for reasons outside of the control of brick workers) and then workers must return home empty-handed. This state of being in a deficit of your debts is called *tutti*.

Most existing qualitative research on brick kiln employment has focused on the social relation of debt, holding debt to be the primary relationship constituting unfree labour in the brick kiln.[6,7,8,9] There has been inadequate examination however of the operation of the everyday labour regime, especially in relation to spaces of living, social relations, and rhythms of work, within the brick kiln itself. An exception to this include Shah's work understanding kilns within West Bengal as a lived space to where Adivasi youth from Jharkhand migrate not only for economic reasons but also to gain independence from their parents and live out prohibited amorous relationships.[10] Similarly, Natarajan et al. show migrant workers' understanding of brick kilns of Cambodia as temporary sites of oppressive work to be endured while building towards durable futures elsewhere, through investments into agrarian livelihoods in rural hometowns.[11] In my previous work, I looked at everyday labouring processes in brick kilns of Khanda as being constituted through changing local political ecological relations of soil extraction and commodification.[12] Also in a different paper, I drew upon kiln workers' life histories of employment within various other informal employment jobs to juxtapose working conditions within these alternate jobs against conditions of work and life in the brick kilns and further understand the reasons for which workers move into and out of kiln employment.[13]

Understanding the negotiation of the COVID-19 crisis, among other critical moments, also requires an understanding of the everyday material practices and social relations by which workers constitute the kiln social space. Brick moulders, for example, live within the kilns in temporary, bare structures called *jhuggis* that they construct out of unbaked mud bricks and are roofed by corrugated metal sheets and tarpaulins in one or two days after arriving. The jhuggis are usually adjacent to the *pashaar* or the flat patch of land allocated to each moulding household where the bricks are moulded and laid to dry. Their jhuggi and pashaar constitute the operational habitation space for every brick moulding household, where they spend most of their time. Life in the brick kilns is marked not only by low wages but also by material scarcity where families must make do with the lack of adequate living space and electricity, lack of basic furniture, and very limited everyday items. Every material object that they possess is used heavily and often through creative repurposing, as families adapt to material scarcity. Workers often have to self-provision for basic needs such as firewood by collecting it from far-off woodlands or must bear deductions to their wage if supplied by the owner or labour contractor. The brick kiln is also a vibrant commercial space for several travelling traders selling bric-a-brac, vegetables, and confectionaries, and workers are highly dependent upon just-in-time purchases from them. The local commerce in brick kilns not only is limited to goods but also involves local youth masquerading as quack doctors who travel through the different kilns soliciting unwell workers. Finally, brick kilns in Khanda also have small shack-shops called *pathaai dukaan* (named for the primary customers being brick moulders) which sell groceries and, more importantly, alcohol to brick kiln workers on credit arrangements.

9.4 The Dismal Work Season of 2019–2020

9.4.1 Experience of the Air Pollution Ban

> 'Pichle saal mein koi nikas nahi hua. Hamesha tutti par. Iss saal bhi wahi hoga. Yeh zameen hi kharaab hai'.
>
> —Rambabu, brick moulder

(Last year as well, we had no take-home wage from the season. We are always in deficit. It seems it will happen this year again. This is a cursed land.)

This section describes how the 2019–2020 work season (usually from October 2019 to June 2020), which was rendered exceptional because of the COVID first lockdown towards the later end of the season (from March 24), can be seen as less exceptional with regard to both previous brick kiln work seasons and a continuation of crisis within the same work season itself.

Rambabu's statement is from December 2019, and he is complaining about the *zameen* or land of Sonipat being unlucky or cursed. He had been coming to Sonipat for the last two years, having worked in kilns in Punjab and other states before, and had faced losses in both these years. The loss here refers to not a loss of capital invested on his part but the investment of labour (as well as of the self since labour is always embodied and inseparable) in migrating and staying at the brick kilns and returning empty-handed (without *nikas*) at the end of the season. This prospect called *tutti* or 'deficit' is produced out of the debt bondage system and the piece-rate wage arrangement where workers are not able to make enough bricks to repay the initial debt (*peshgi*) and accruing *kharchas* by the end of the season.[14] Rambabu's statement marks that he had experienced *tutti* in the previous work season in another brick kiln at Khanda and the anticipation that this year would be the same.

'We eat a lot of potatoes now. We bought an *allu ka katta* (sack of potatoes) of 25 kilos, and it will last us 2 *pandrahi* (2 fortnights). We cannot afford a lot of raw vegetables now, so we are getting by with eating stuffed rotis or alu sabzi (potato curry)'—Manoj, brick moulder.

Manoj's description of his family's predicament is from an interview conducted in November 2019. Together with Rambabu's quote, it also marks the early work season of 2019–2020 as a period of profound crisis for kiln workers. Manoj had arrived with his family in September and had yet to mould many bricks to add to their account, against their debt, when they were hit by closure of the kilns. The owner had stopped supplying soil to mould bricks with, and workers like Manoj were sitting idle. In response to two months of idleness, Manoj anticipated that they would go into *tutti* and hence guarded against that possibility by cutting consumption expenditure from already very moderate levels.

This crisis was caused by the enforcement of the brick kiln burning ban in response to high levels of air pollution in Delhi-NCR. The Graded Response

Action Plan (GRAP), a measure put in place to tackle air pollution, comes into effect when the atmospheric concentration of PM 2.5 or PM 10 particles in Delhi-NCR exceeds a determined level and mandates strict curbs on industrial emissions including a ban on firing in any brick kiln oven within Delhi-NCR.[15] While the GRAP's mandated measures are predictable considering the annual recurrence of Delhi's smog season during winters, what was unpredictable was the actual enforcement of these measures in 2019. Within my first fieldwork period in the winter of 2018, many brick kilns continued to be fired despite the ban being in place and only stopped firing for a few days around Diwali when both levels of pollution and national attention to the pollution crisis peaked. In 2019, however, there was much more stringent enforcement from Pollution Control Board officials through surprise inspections and hefty fines which effectively shut operations down all over Khanda. This enforcement caught kiln owners as well as workers who had already migrated into the kilns as they were unaware of the enforcement. While kiln owners suffered losses, which were also partially offset through price of bricks in their inventory going up against scarcity of bricks in market, the ban was felt much more devastatingly by workers who could not make bricks through the whole four months (until 31st January) during which the ban was in place. The idle time was felt not just as the loss in income but as accumulation of debt and a dimming of the hope for taking back any money to Bihar for the off-season period between June and October. Several workers who were single men fled the kilns for other jobs.[16] It was mostly the workers who had families and had made substantial investments into migrating to the kilns, and had fewer opportunities available of adequately remunerative work, who stayed in the kilns and hoped for brick making to restart.

The ban period was experienced as also a struggle to manage everyday expenses for kiln workers, despite the consumption cutbacks that Manoj described. Under the usual arrangement, workers' wages are held back until the end of the season, and each household is instead paid an allowance or *kharcha* every fortnight to manage routine expenses. The kharcha differs according to the family size but is often barely adequate to meet expenses, as owners use the kharcha to incentivize production, raising kharcha for households making more bricks. This act is justified through an argument of workers not being able to responsibly manage their expenditure, especially men being prone to wasting their wages on alcohol otherwise. During the ban, this paternalist logic was extended to reduce kharcha even further and push workers to the brink of a reproduction crisis. In reality, the kharcha was reduced to minimize the exposure of owners in case workers fled the kilns which was rife during this period.

What the reduced kharcha did was also to make workers' everyday purchases more expensive as they got caught in debt traps with the small grocery and alcohol vending shops (locally called *pathaai dukaan* or moulders' shops). When allowances are low, it is not worthwhile for the worker to travel to the larger *mandi* or market in Kharkhoda where items are cheaper. Instead, workers have to buy under shop credit arrangements with these pathaai shops where every item's price is marked up. These small one-roomed establishments located next to the brick kilns are run by local villagers and they sell to kiln workers on a shop-credit basis.

In the kiln where Manoj worked, the pathaai shop is run by the younger son of the farmer on whose leased land the brick kiln is operating, while the farmer's elder son works as a Munshi (accountant-cum-manager) in the kiln. The kharcha of barely Rs. 1,500–2,000 to manage his family of six for a fortnight was inadequate and Manoj had to rely on shop-credit from the pathaai shop to make ends meet. By December, the shopkeeper had three months of credit pending with workers and decided to stop selling goods on credit anymore while recovering cash out from workers' allowances. Manoj received Rs. 2,000 and the shopkeeper took away Rs. 1,300 of it, while refusing to offer any credit. In my final days of fieldwork, I witnessed Manoj quarrelling with the shopkeeper and his brother, the Munshi, angrily shouting at them that his children would go hungry unless the shopkeeper gave goods on credit. Caught at the intersection of the bonded labour wage relation, spatial immobility, exploitative owners, and extractive shopkeepers, workers like Manoj were already in a state of crisis before COVID-19 affected the work season.

9.5 The Immediate Aftermath of the Pandemic (March–July 2020)

As mentioned, from a contagion standpoint, the pandemic did not have devastating consequences in the brick kilns in Khanda. The brick kilns functioned as settlements that were cut off from the local village, and only limited flows of villagers and commerce continued between them. Indeed, as we see later, the Sarpanch of Khanda disallowed workers from coming into the village settlement during the first lockdown, other than using the main road.

Work in the brick kilns was not directly stopped for the imposition of lockdown but due to disruptions in the supply of production material. Coal, the supply of which to brick kiln can be precarious in regular times, ran out very soon and stopped the baking of bricks. Some owners resorted to changing the fuel mixture from coal to locally sourced *tudi* or mustard stalks even if it led to bricks of lower strength. As during the air pollution crisis, the salaries of firemen and truck drivers were cut in half.

The work of moulding went on for some time as sundried bricks can be stored for later burning by arranging them as a circular structure called a *chatta* (up to 10,000 bricks in a single chatta) and then covering with a plastic sheet for the rain. This is however limited by the available free space within the kiln area and the owners' strategy on the quantity of inventory. Moulding however also stopped in several places when sand (ensures wet bricks don't stick to the mould or the ground) being bought from other villages ran out. Moulders were visiting each other's pashaar to ask if they had surplus sand so that they could take in sacks to continue working.

For a majority of the lockdown period in 2020, piece-rate workers sat idle as before. However, this period of idleness was viewed differently as the possibilities of earning wages had shrunk. As Prabhu, another moulder, told me, 'This year, everyone has tutti. But this is not concerning as no one will flee (the kiln). Many people are saying they will just stay here through the *choumasa* and do some other work (the monsoons months which is the off-season of kiln work)'. Karu stated that because in the light of the exodus of migrant workers and the crisis within other worksites, brick kilns in Khanda manifested as a refuge albeit a very sinadequate one. For one, brick kiln workers had food and housing security during the crisis. The concentration of thousands of migrant workers in Khanda gave easy visibility for the district administration who instructed brick kiln owners to make sure of food and basic supplies to workers. As a result, several relatives of brick kiln workers who worked in Delhi-NCR and had been affected by job losses or faced eviction from inability to pay rent walked to Khanda to stay in the brick kiln. In a previous paper, I had pointed brick kilns to be a key site within translocal householding strategies for migrant workers.[17],[18] While brick kiln employment offers married middle-aged workers an opportunity to stay with their family and keep children close, there is proportionately much less presence of single young men between the age of 18 and 30 in the kilns. Unmarried young men who may have grown up in different brick kiln sites take every opportunity to exit the confines of kiln work and enter into other forms of 'factory work' or jobs in the urban informal sector that are considered more aspirational and respectable than moulding. This is why there was a stream of young male workers who re-joined their families in the brick kilns during the pandemic. For instance, both the son and nephew of one brick moulder walked to Khanda after the belt-making factory in Sonipat they were working in was closed down. There is also no one, to my knowledge, who left from Khanda to undertake the arduous journey of walking back to their far-off hometowns, as we saw thousands of migrant workers do during the tragic exodus. A group of moulders from Aligarh in Western Uttar Pradesh did try this. They left Khanda at 10 AM but were stopped and turned back at the Delhi-Sonipat border by the police, returning to Khanda at 2 AM that night.

In the initial phase, instead of relying on the shops, owners were supplying dry rations to the workers. Their vehicles had been granted permission as supply vehicles so they could cross state boundaries (between Delhi and Sonipat) unimpeded. However, the dry ration was still being deducted from wage, that too at an expensive rate. For the 25 kg sack of rice that workers would get normally at Rs 500 from Kharkhoda market, Rs 750 was deducted from workers' wages.

The key reproductive crisis during the initial lockdown was however felt not in the absence of food but in the shortage of firewood. Access to firewood is anyway an ongoing problem for workers in Khanda where there is not much easily accessible firewood and there is too much demand from villagers and kiln workers alike. In many kilns, the arrangement was for the labour contractor to supply firewood purchased from traders but that stopped with the pandemic. Workers initially resorted to buying *upla* or dried cow dung cakes from women in the village or travelling to the public land around an irrigation canal 2.5 km from Khanda with their wheelbarrows to collect firewood. Both these means were however soon curtailed as the Sarpanch of Khanda, as a public health measure, disallowed workers from coming into the village settlement or using the main road to reach the canal. The deficit in firewood was resolved through workers rationing their supply and borrowing from each other, through the owner paying farmers for the right to collect firewood from their fields or from workers surreptitiously collecting from neighbouring fields at night.

The lack of access to *khaini* (chewing tobacco) and alcohol also was a problem for kiln workers. Brick kiln worksites are notorious for the availability of alcohol and drunkenness. The pathaai shops offer alcohol on credit throughout the year. Alcohol and khaini were either unavailable or priced prohibitively high during the lockdown. The Rs 5 packet of khaini was selling for Rs.110, and addicted workers were still buying it, making do with a packet for seven to eight days that would be consumed twice a day. The same was true for country alcohol selling at Rs 500 a bottle instead of Rs 135. In one instance, as the kiln workers made a direct deal with a khaini distributor to purchase packets in bulk, the distributor was threatened by the pathaai shopkeepers to keep away, a way to protect their high profits during COVID.

The brick kiln season of 2019–2020 ended in July as workers left the kilns on buses hired by the owner after the relaxation of lockdown norms. All the workers I know of returned empty-handed after making very few bricks throughout the season and mostly sitting idle. Having a direct bus from Delhi to their home district in Bihar is generally too expensive for workers who have to use the crowded trains instead. A worker I spoke to in 2022 said they were considering this year to rent a bus at Rs 1,300 per worker instead of the train, as the travel back by bus in the COVID year was quite convenient for them.

9.6 The Interpretations of the Pandemic Within the Brick Kilns

Brick kilns are often relatively isolated in their location within village farmlands, at a distance from the main settlement as well as major roads. The lockdown exacerbated this isolation as it dramatically reduced the flow of people and commerce between the village and the kilns. Further only a few days into the first lockdown, the Sarpanch (or village head) restricted kiln workers from entering the village settlement areas even to purchase fuelwood or cow dung cakes from households (the village shops were closed). Alongside isolation, brick kiln workers' orientation to the virus was also influenced by their abject state of illiteracy. Migrant brick kiln workers are deprived of school education for their children, and as brick kiln migration is intergenerational among marginalized communities, so is illiteracy.[19] A large proportion of moulders in Khanda belong to the *Musahar* caste from Bihar, a community whose literacy rate in Bihar in 2018 was just 29%.[20]

Illiteracy and isolation however can hardly be singled out as drivers of irrational thinking around the COVID-19 virus given how conspiracy theories and alternative medicine often featured in the global cultural response to the pandemic, even among world leaders. The interpretations of the pandemic among kiln workers were drawn from their traditional and spiritual worldviews, experience of diseases, and information (including misinformation) from different sources, including the internet, to make sense of the COVID-19 virus. These interpretations differed among brick kiln workers, especially those from different caste backgrounds and regions, as workers expressed varying mixtures of fear, doubt, and denial of the threat of the virus. Laxman, a Musahar worker from Navada, Bihar, asked me over the phone how a disease originating from a bat could affect them when they have been eating bat meat for many years in their village. Within their traditional medicine as well, they put bat blood in the ear to relieve ear pain.

Ajay, another worker of the Musahar caste, stated that most of the moulders in his kiln have stopped working at night from fear of COVID-19. This was especially intuitive since from the month of March onwards, brick kiln workers work late into the night (until 3 AM) in order to rest through the hot afternoons. After hearing of the proclamations for *Thali bajao* (Bang utensils) and *Diya jalao* (light earthen lamps) from the Indian Prime Minister Narendra Modi in his televised address, the workers became convinced that COVID must be a ghostly entity as these actions are culturally associated with warding off evil spirits. Despite the attempts of the owner and Munshis to persuade them otherwise, some workers persisted with this belief and refused to work at night, even at a loss to their income. Such a consequence that affected the incomes of low-waged workers highlight how the worldviews of workers avoidant and reverential of evil natural forces differed from some nationalist representations of COVID-19. Kaur and Ramaswamy (2020) demonstrated how the COVID-19 virus was reimagined in popular depictions as a demonic force to be vanquished by a capable nationalist and religious figure, donning a stethoscope and protecting Bhārat Mātā (Mother India).[21]

Another factor that conditioned kiln workers' response to the virus is also the wide gap in access to qualified and affordable healthcare services for which kiln workers are completely dependent on unqualified healthcare providers, mostly youth from nearby villages. The glaring absence of healthcare infrastructure also means that basic messages around pandemic awareness never reach the kilns. The disregard for health warning also continued in a later pandemic scare, the outbreak of Avian Influenza (H5N8) or Bird Flu in Haryana in January and February 2021. During this time, when hundreds of thousands of birds were being culled across the state, some poultry owners and traders were selling live hens for as cheap as Rs 20 for a hen (what would be Rs 150 otherwise). The shopkeepers themselves wouldn't touch the hen while selling. For the whole of that month, brick kiln workers would buy several birds at a time and eat chicken every day.

9.7 Conclusion

As the foreword of this book suggests, there can be no universalising narrative of the pandemic. COVID upended the lives of migrant workers in dramatic and tragic ways, most visibly represented in the great exodus from Indian cities. The brick kilns in Khanda represent a different form of the tragic impact of the virus. Here, workers with families could not afford to make the thousand-kilometre journey back home even if they wished to. Unlike cities where employers and landlords could stop wage payments and drive workers out, brick kiln workers in Khanda lived in a prominent migration cluster and were therefore visible to the local administration. This ensured that workers could access basic necessities of food and shelter through kiln owners. However, the gaze of the state did not extend to protecting wages, and workers experienced the lockdown as a period of idle wagelessness and accumulating debts. In narrating the COVID-19 lockdown, workers would emphasize the anxiety of debts and cutdowns in basic reproductive consumption as central to their experience over the fear of disease. This anxiety appeared continuous to them for the entire 2019–2020 work season which began with the stringent air pollution ban, followed by frequent work stoppages from itinerant rainfall and culminated with the COVID lockdown.

The chapter reflects the narrative presented by workers in understanding how workers negotiated the pandemic. My analysis resonates with the claim in this book that grief and trauma marked the experience of COVID-19 for marginal migrant workers much more than the strangeness of COVID. The chapter described in detail the two events of the 2019–2020 work season (the air pollution ban and the lockdown) in conjunction and juxtaposed these anomalous situations, both of which created acute livelihood shocks, against the structural conditions of work in the kilns. These conditions of brick kiln work including debt bondage, low wages paid at piece rate and the absence of any form of social security, among others, are deeply exploitative and enable capitalist owners to transfer risk from eventualities such as COVID-19 or factory bans to affect workers' wages and living conditions. The continuities of the lockdown crisis with other anomalous events as well as with precarious life more generally circumscribe hope that the lockdown may produce new political subjectivities among workers towards demanding greater labour rights, even in the face of existential challenges.

Notes

1 Delhi-NCR or the Delhi-National Capital Region is a planning region marking the urban agglomeration around Delhi which includes neighbouring Sonipat district where Khanda village is located.

2 Pratik Mishra, The making of urban peripheries and peripheral labor: Brick kilns and circular migration in and beyond greater Delhi, *South Asia Multidisciplinary Academic Journal* 26 (2021). https://doi.org/10.4000/samaj.7276. See for how this is a common translocal householding pattern for kiln families.
3 Janet Roitman, *Anti-Crisis*, Durham, NC: Duke University Press, 2013: 176.
4 Shailendra Kumar, and Sanghamitra Choudhury, Migrant workers and human rights: A critical study on India's Covid-19 lockdown policy, *Social Sciences & Humanities Open* 3 (2021): 100130.
5 Pratik Mishra, Surplus population in-situ: Brick kiln labor and the production of idle time, *Focaal Journal* 97 (2023): 49–62. https://doi.org/10.3167/fcl.2023.970105. See the politics of idle time for a detailed discussion.
6 Isabelle Guérin, and Govindan Venkatasubramanian, The socio-economy of debt. Revisiting debt bondage in times of financialization, *Geoforum* 37 (2022): 174–84. https://doi.org/10.1016/j.geoforum.2020.05.020.
7 Jan Breman, *Footloose Labour: Working in India's Informal Economy*, Cambridge University Press, 1996.
8 Sunita Kumari, Neo-bondage in the brick kiln industry: A case study of Bihar, *Social Change* 48 (3) (2018): 384–97. https://doi.org/10.1177/0049085718781687.
9 Komal Chauhan, Why do Dalits Migrate? A case study of neo-bondage in Western Uttar Pradesh, *Contemporary Voice of Dalit* 14 (1) (2022): 95–102. https://doi.org/10.1177/2455328X211042500.
10 Alpa Shah, The labour of love: Seasonal migration from Jharkhand to the brick kilns of other states in India, *Contributions to Indian Sociology* 40 (1) (2006): 91–118. https://doi.org/10.1177/006996670504000104.
11 Nitya Natarajan, Laurie Parsons, and Katherine Brickell, Debt-bonded brick kiln workers and their intent to return: Towards a labour geography of smallholder farming persistence in Cambodia, *Antipode* 51 (5) (2019): 1581–99. https://doi.org/10.1111/anti.12564.
12 Pratik Mishra, Urbanisation through brick kilns: The interrelationship between appropriation of nature and labour regimes, *Urbanisation* 5 (1) (2020): 17–36.
13 Mishra, The making of urban peripheries and peripheral labor.
14 While workers may be in debt to the owner at the end of the season, the debt would not be transferred across two work seasons and the debt would be wiped as workers leave empty-handed with return travel expected to be paid by employers. This seems to be the standard for brick kilns in North India and at least for my region. The practice of trapping workers under debt across work seasons was still a feature of bonded labour in brick kilns until the 1980s in Delhi (BBMSS 19) and only later removed through a mix of market forces, enforcement of law against bonded labour, and labour movements.
15 What is GRAP and what it suggests for each pollution category, *The Indian Express*, 14 November 2021. Accessed 26 June 2024. https://indianexpress.com/article/cities/delhi/what-is-grap-and-what-it-suggests-for-each-pollution-category-7621972/.
16 The debt owed by workers to kiln owners and labour contractors, though illegal, does incarcerate workers to an extent as they run the risk of being beaten if they are caught trying to flee the kiln. However, the open space of the kiln presents little opportunity for owners or contractors to effectively stop workers who generally flee in the middle of the night and manage to arrange transportation.
17 Mishra, The making of urban peripheries and peripheral labor.
18 Priti Ramamurthy, Translocal householding, *Comparative Studies of South Asia, Africa and the Middle East* 40 (1) (2020): 86–94.
19 Pratik Mishra, What financial literacy among brick kiln workers says about India's education system, *The Wire*, 23 September 2020. Accessed 26 June 2024.

https://thewire.in/education/what-financial-literacy-among-brick-kiln-workers-says-about-indias-education-system.

20 Government of India. *Handbook of Social Welfare Statistics*, New Delhi: Ministry of Social Justice and Empowerment, 2018. Accessed 26 June 2024. https://socialjustice.nic.in/writereaddata/UploadFile/HANDBOOKSocialWelfareStatistice2018.pdf.

21 Ravinder Kaur, and Sumathi Ramaswamy, The goddess and the virus in Vinayak Chaturvedi (ed.), *The Pandemic: Perspectives on Asia*, Ann Arbor, MI: The Association for Asian Studies, 2020: 75–94.

10 Community Resilience in the Western Himalayas

Lessons from the Pandemic

Ritwika Patgiri

10.1 Introduction

Mountains are one of the earliest indicators of climate change. They are home to 1.2 billion people of the world and a source of drinking water, irrigation, and hydroelectricity for as many as 40% of the world's population. Mountain ecosystems are more sensitive to climate change and there is evidence of them being affected at a faster rate than terrestrial habitats (Henrik Terbek 2014). This in turn could have severe consequences for water provision and livelihoods in downstream regions.

The Indian Himalayan Region (IHR) is a massive climate change hotspot and is projected to experience the most severe effects of climate change outside the poles (Gergan 2016). The IHR can be divided into three broad regions: (i) Western Himalayan Region, (ii) Eastern Himalayan Region, and (iii) Central Himalayan Region. The Western Himalayan Region (Uttarakhand, Himachal Pradesh (HP), Ladakh, and Jammu and Kashmir) is the largest region of the Indian Himalayas and is alone home to around 51 million people and many diverse forms of flora and fauna. This region is also a major source of water for the rest of the country and the mountain springs serve as the primary source of water for rural villages in the region.

The COVID-19 pandemic exposed the vulnerabilities of the region and the state machinery. A few months after the economic lockdown of India, poverty levels in the country returned to the 2016 levels. Three percent of the Indian labour force lost their jobs while many others suffered economic and health setbacks (Rahman and Pingali 2024). An exogenous shock of such a large scale leads to the loss of income and livelihood and pushes people into destitution. While some people were able to successfully escape poverty, the pandemic increased the vulnerabilities of the marginalized and poorer sections of the society. The Western Himalayan states of India had witnessed depopulation and the emergence of ghost villages prior to the pandemic. The lockdown, however, gave rise to a trend of reverse migration. Tourism, one of the largest livelihood generating sectors in the region after agriculture, came to an instant halt. Young people lost their livelihoods in large numbers. While the pandemic reflected the abysmal state of public health of the region, what

DOI: 10.4324/9781003591641-14

also became evident was the failure of the state to accommodate the returnee migrants and the young people who had lost their livelihoods in one of the most vulnerable regions in the world, which further exacerbated the region's challenges.

Traditional cultures often saw voluntary charitable assistance to the needy, motivated by either religious or moral or social values. During times of scarcity and famine, there are instances of Egyptian and Roman rulers distributing free food to the people during the imperial era. This was mostly done to ensure peace, avoid civil unrest, and maintain law and order. With the emergence of nation-states and democratic governments, the provision of social security and social protection is seen as a social contract, providing the state the legitimacy to govern its citizens (Rahman and Pingali 2024). The COVID-19 pandemic exposed the weak and fractured nature of such commitments of the state, which was particularly evident when images and videos of millions of migrants trying to walk back to their native places emerged. The Western Himalayan states saw a surge of return migrants during the period. This chapter attempts to understand how community resilience emerged as a form of response to the pandemic at a time when the state failed to intervene. This chapter focuses on how the COVID-19 pandemic has affected the lives of people living in a region battling climate change, water crisis, and natural disasters in the midst of the pandemic and how the communities have responded to these challenges.

It is important to note that the Western Himalayan region is not a homogeneous region in terms of social demography and economic factors. However, the region faces many similar vagaries of nature and human interference (Das and Meher 2019). Several studies have noted the various climate-related disasters that the region faces including cloudburst, thunderstorm, glacial lake outburst flood, and forest fires (Dimri et al. 2017). The dangers of defining an area of study cannot be underestimated. As Alan Everitt (1977), a British local historian noted that the boundaries of a historical region will vary according to whether we are thinking of a regional landscape or a regional society. It shall also vary according to whether we are thinking of a farming region, a social neighbourhood, a country community, or an industrial region. The justification behind using the Western Himalayan region for this study, apart from the similar impact of climate change and geographical similarities, can also be understood in its historical patterns in agriculture, trends in tourism, and employment structure. Further, both Himachal Pradesh and Uttarakhand have the highest propensity of male out-migration in India and both the states, along with Ladakh, saw a huge number of return migrants during the pandemic-ensued lockdown. Along with climate change vulnerabilities, the region was exposed to an unprecedented rise in people. Accommodating the return migrants became a major challenge for the region.

This chapter is divided into five sections. Section 10.2 describes the economy of the Western Himalayan region. More than 50% of the population in all the states of the region are dependent on agriculture and at least 4% are engaged in tourism-related activities (transportation, accommodation, and food). Out-migration is an important phenomenon in the region, which is driven by several factors including lack of employment opportunities and climate-related issues like water scarcity, rise in natural hazards, and degradation of land and other natural resources. This has led to an emergence of *ghost villages* in many areas of the region. The third section shows the impact of the pandemic in the region. As the country witnessed a nationwide lockdown, the region saw the return of many migrants. Accommodating the returnees and generating employment became the most crucial tasks for the economy. The section also discusses the role of the state and social security during the crisis. Finally, the last section looks at how community resilience emerged in the region as a form of coping mechanism because of the pandemic through narratives.

When disasters occur, no two communities are likely to experience the same event exactly the same way. Thus, community resilience literature has always focused at the local level (Longstaff et al. 2010). Local emergency planning and response activities are often guided by five interrelated community sub-systems—ecology, economy, physical infrastructure, civil society, and governance. This study tried to understand the local economy and its problems, and further focus on why certain resilience techniques can work.

10.2 State of the Western Himalayan Economy and Climate

Agriculture is the dominant source of income and employment in the Western Himalayan region of India. About 90% of the population in Himachal Pradesh live in rural areas as 62% of the total workers are engaged in farm-based activities (Asian Development Bank 2010). The communities here predominantly rely on agriculture, leaving approximately 80% of the residents to depend on rainfall for their livelihoods (Loria and Bhardwaj 2016). In Uttarakhand, over 70% of the population is dependent on agriculture as the chief livelihood source. However, the share of agriculture has been falling in the region like the rest of the country and its contribution to the economy is the lowest amongst all the three sectors.

Hilly states are characterized by small land holdings, low population density, traditional farming practices, and high dependence on natural resources. Data shows that more than 90% of the population in hilly regions earn their livelihood from agriculture and other farm-related activities. Previous studies on the region have similarly shown that the region's economy is mainly dependent on natural resources and agricultural support land, especially, plays a role in the household economy (Singh 1993).

The region has witnessed a transformation from agriculture to services. In Himachal Pradesh, agriculture contributes 9.4% of the net state domestic product while services contribute 43.48%. The share of primary sectors which include agriculture, forestry, fishing, and mining and quarrying has declined from 35.52% in 1990–91 to 16.01% during 2016–17 and to 14.58% during

Table 10.1 Share of various sectors in state GDP as of 2019–20

State/Region	*Share of Agriculture*	*Share of Manufacturing*	*Share of Services*
Uttarakhand	9.40%	44.85%	37.94%
Himachal Pradesh	14.58%	41.94%	43.48%
Jammu and Kashmir	31.7%	10%	58.3%
India	16.5%	29.5%	55.3%

2019–20 in Himachal. In Uttarakhand, agriculture contributes around 10% to state gross domestic product (GDP) and services contribute 38%.

In terms of employment, the 2022–23 Periodic Labour Force Survey data shows that the share of agriculture in Himachal is 62% and about 58% in Uttarakhand. The share of agriculture in employment in Jammu and Kashmir and Ladakh is around 51%. Hence, agriculture remains the most important source of occupation for more than half of the region's population. Other than construction and manufacturing, transportation, food, and accommodation are other important sources of employment in the region.

Tourism, which is a part of the service sector and includes the sectors of transport, food, and accommodation, is one of the fastest growing sectors in the region. In Uttarakhand, tourism contributes about 4.4% to the state GDP and employs 2% of the population. Similarly, the contribution of tourism to the Himachal economy is about 7% in 2019–20 (India Brand Equity Foundation 2022). While industries like pharmaceuticals play important contribution to the economy of the state, the domestic tourist inflow in the state has reached 5.63 million in 2021.

An analysis of the trend of domestic and foreign tourist inflows in the region shows that there is a fall in tourist inflow during the pandemic.

Table 10.2 shows how both domestic and international tourist inflows have changed in the region from 2002 to 2021. Uttarakhand has seen a significant rise in the growth of domestic tourists from 2004 to 2009, which came down in 2020 with the advent of the pandemic.

A look at the absolute numbers from Figure 10.1 shows that the tourist inflow in Uttarakhand saw a rise till the pandemic. The post-pandemic growth has not yet reached its previous high in the state.

Similarly, for Himachal Pradesh and Jammu and Kashmir, the post-pandemic rise in both domestic and international tourist inflow is yet to reach the previous highs (as seen from Figures 10.2 and 10.3).

We also take a comparative look at both domestic and international tourists in all the three states of the region. Uttarakhand (as seen from Figure 10.4) has seen the highest inflow of tourists in both pre- and post-pandemic years, whereas Himachal has seen the lowest inflow of tourists post-pandemic.

The drastic fall in tourist inflows in the region because of the pandemic had a heavy impact on the local economy. The pandemic forced lakhs of

Table 10.2 State-wise domestic and foreign tourist visits growth percentage

Year	*2002–03*		*2003–04*		*2004–09*		*2009–10*		*2010–20*		*2020–21*	
State/Region	*Domestic*	*International*	*Domestic*	*International*	*Domestic*	*International*	*Domestic*	*International*	*Domestic*	*International*	*Domestic*	*International*
Himachal	11.8	16.3	14.5	21.7	73.9	96.0	16.6	13.2	-75.4	-90.6	77.6	-88.4
Uttarakhand	2.2	22.5	8.2	13.9	87.1	69.3	37.7	19.5	-76.8	-67.5	177.4	-79.4
Jammu and Kashmir	25.8	211.1	19.7	65.4	34.2	35.4	8.0	-11.7	-74.7	-88.9	349.1	-69.0

Source: India Tourism Statistics (Ministry of Tourism, Government of India)

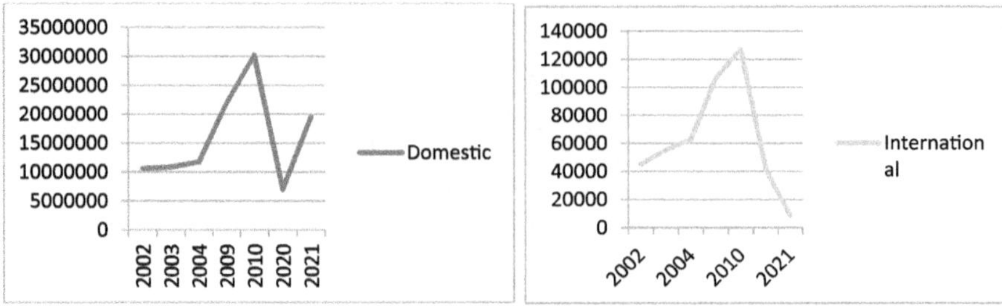

Figure 10.1 Domestic and international tourist flows in Uttarakhand

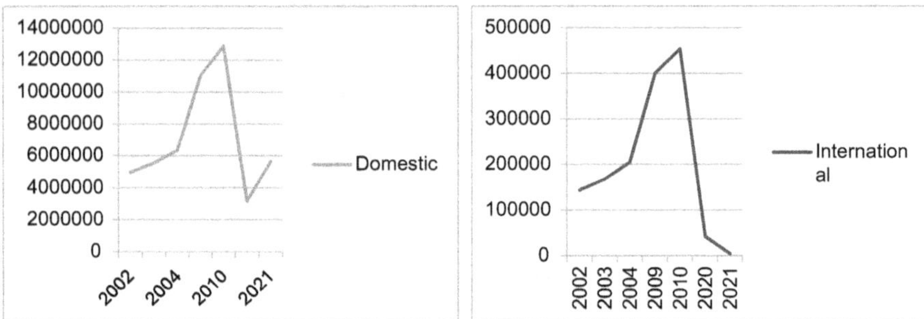

Figure 10.2 Domestic and international tourist flows in Himachal

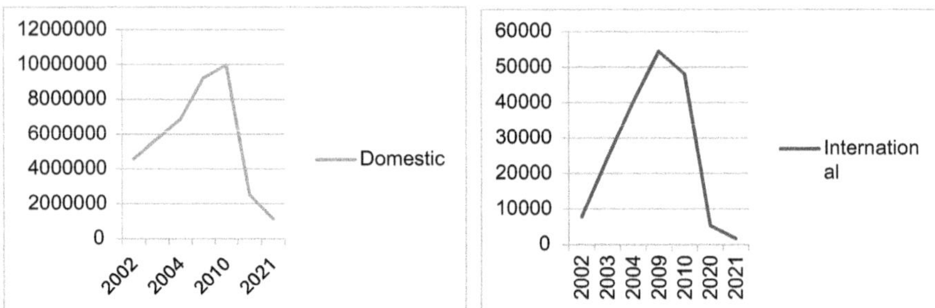

Figure 10.3 Domestic and international tourist flows in Jammu and Kashmir

people of the region who are dependent on the tourism and hospitality industry to the brink of loss of livelihood. An estimated 3.8 crore people have been unemployed which is translated to 70% of the entire workforce from the Indian tourism and hospitality sector (PTI 2020).

The story of the Western Himalayan economy cannot be complete without the mention of the migration patterns in the region. The Western Himalayan region has witnessed a high rate of migration. Especially in Uttarakhand,

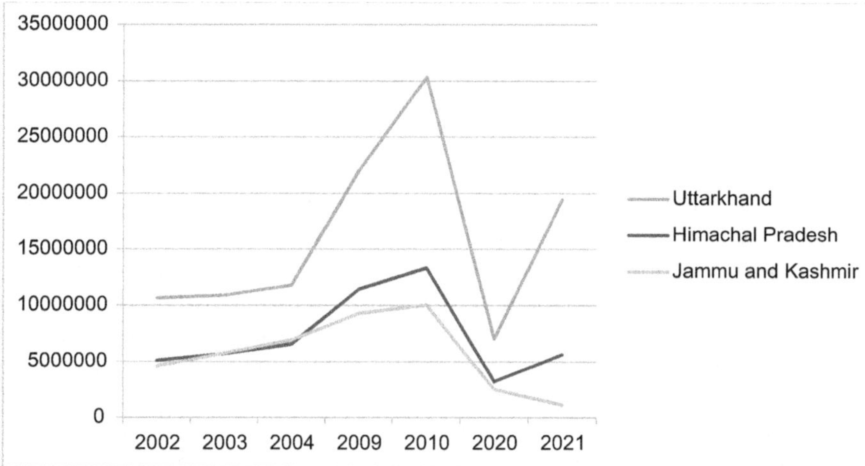

Figure 10.4 Domestic and international tourists in the Western Himalayas

there is a difference in population growth in hill districts and plain districts. According to data from the 2011 Census, the overall population growth in Uttarakhand was 1.7% but this differed significantly for plain and hill districts. The growth rate of population in plains was 2.8%, while the growth rate in hill districts was 0.7%, which is one-fourth of the population growth in plain districts. This huge difference in the two types of districts is indicative that there is huge emigration from the hill districts. The major reasons for emigration from mountain regions to other areas are the dependence of subsistence economy, a lack of sufficient local employment opportunities, and search of livelihood opportunities. Emigration from the region has led to significant depopulation in the region and subsequently, a rise in "ghost villages."

Migration has always been a livelihood diversification strategy for most people in the Hindu Kush Himalayan region. Recent literature has found that around 65% of the 210 million people in this region suffer from malnutrition, perpetual food insecurity, degradation of natural resources, and frequent disasters that threaten the livelihood security of the people of the region. In this context, migration is seen as an effective strategy for livelihood that can help alleviate poverty in mountain areas.

When I spoke to one of the workers who had migrated to Bihar from Ladakh, he told me that he had lost all his crops to monsoon flood and there was no other alternative for him. Many migrants like Nado[1] cannot continue farming in their region to earn livelihood because of flooding and other climate change-induced changes, leaving them with no option but to migrate out. Studies have found that global warming in the Himalayan region has started affecting farming and other livelihoods in the hydropower sector and will cause floods downstream.

Another reason for migration is water scarcity in the region which is aggravated by climate change in the region. Water scarcity is often understood in terms of volumetric deficit which often ignores how resource appropriation is done by the decisive and the elite on one hand, and how collective action around scarce resources is carried out on the other (Mehta 2011; Shah 2023). Studies have documented that scarcity can be differentiated based on geographical location and social class (Badiger et al. 2014). The translation of availability of physical water into its accessibility is often dependent on the current state, scale, and ability of water infrastructure and institutions to overcome seasonal changes and reduce the water burden (Shah and Badiger 2020). A major part of drinking water supply in the mountainous parts of Uttarakhand is spring based and in Himachal Pradesh, a majority of the people rely on traditional sources for drinking and irrigation. According to estimates by the NITI Aayog, there are about five million springs across India and close to three million of them are in the Indian Himalayan Region, including the Eastern Himalayas, more than half of which have been estimated to have dried up or have become seasonal, resulting in acute water shortage across the region. Shah and Badiger (2020), in the context of the Eastern Himalayas, have argued that water crisis in the region is a result of a conundrum created by interlinked problems across political unwillingness, insufficient investments, failure of cooperation between the State and the regional institutions, and inadequacies in local governance including institutional capacity.

As agriculture has become difficult to pursue along with water shortages, migration has become a common phenomenon in the region. When the Uttarakhand Rural Development and Migration Commission (URDMC) did a telephonic interview during the lockdown to understand why people migrate from Uttarakhand, apart from reasons like unemployment, health, educational opportunities, and climate change-related issues, small landholding size has also been mentioned by the migrants. It is believed that agriculture with small landholding size is insufficient for the sustenance of the household. According to the same study, Uttarakhand had 1,048 uninhabited villages called ghost villages or *bhutiya gaon* in 2011, which has increased by 735 since then along with abandoned agricultural landscapes across several hill districts of the state. Uttarakhand has been indeed marked by long-duration out-migration even before the COVID-19 pandemic. Mamgain and Reddy (2017) found that 73% of the migration across 18 villages of the state is long-duration migration. Their study also found that 36% of the households surveyed have left their villages permanently. The permanent migration has remained a disturbing feature of Uttarakhand. The migration has been for regular salaried jobs and not for manual work, but most of these jobs are low paid and petty. In fact, Uttarakhand is the second state after Uttar Pradesh to have witnessed large-scale and rapid migration according to the Economic

Survey 2016–17. 35% of the migrations happened after 2000, when the state was formed (Integrated Mountain Initiative 2019).

Further, Sati (2021) found that post-2011, most of the migration in Uttarakhand is internal, from mountainous regions to urban centres within the state. About 734 villages are depopulated, and in 367 villages, the population has decreased by more than 50%. The study found that unemployment is the major problem in rural areas as more than 50% of out-migration occurred for employment.

While 246 people migrated daily according to Integrate Mountain Initiative, 50.16% of the migrations occurred due to no jobs, 15.21% due to lack of education facilities, and 8.83% due to the absence of medical facilities, the Economic Survey 2019–20 said. Some 5.61% of the farmers fled in distress as animals such as monkeys and pigs would regularly invade their farms and destroy standing crop. 3900 villages are presently victims of migration.

The analysis of the Census of 2001–11 reveals that more than 2,26,949 farmer families of Uttarakhand have migrated from their native villages. After the migration, main source of their livelihood, elsewhere, was daily wage labourers mainly in factories and shops. For them life has become more vulnerable. Consequent to migrations, today, only less than 20% agricultural land in the hill districts of Uttarakhand is being farmed and the remaining 80% has become fallow land for varying periods.

10.2.1 Impact of Climate Change in the Region

We have already discussed how climate change-related issues have forced people in the region to emigrate, but there is a need to understand how vulnerable the region is to the effects of the global climate change. Climate change makes regions uninhabitable, unproductive, and unfit for human use due to rising natural disasters like storms, melting glaciers, and changing rainfall patterns (World Bank 2012). Furthermore, climate change can also lead to negative impacts on livelihood and economic opportunities and conflicts over dwindling resources (Wrathall et al. 2013).

Research has found that the Himalayan region is warming by 0.3 degrees Celsius to 0.7 degrees Celsius above the global average leading to a decline in Asia's largest freshwater reserve. Stretching from Afghanistan to Myanmar, the Hindu Kush Himalayan region is a 2,000-mile-long mountain and is home to the world's highest peaks. However, these peaks are warming faster than the rest of the planet. Almost all disasters and hazards of the region have become intensified because of climate change.

Migration, as noted in the previous section, has emerged as a major response to climate change. The research on climate-induced migration broadly talks about two key conclusions—migration as a strategy for adapting to adverse conditions (Bardsley and Hugo 2010) and migration resulting due to a lack of capacity to adapt by the local population (Tacoli 2009). However, the decision to migrate is determined not only by climatic and other factors but also by a range of socio-economic determinants, including socio-economic aspirations and cultural values (Black et al. 2011). Climate-related factors can, in turn, impact socio-economic factors like education, access to health and services, and agricultural income. Migration patterns also differ according to gender, age, caste, and class positions.

Migration as an adaptive strategy can be understood as a form of livelihood resilience which occurs when livelihood systems can no longer absorb stress. Further, the dominant structure influences adaptive migration. In a study based in Honduras, Wrathall et al. (2013) found that apart from the storm-displaced population in a catastrophically flooded village, close to 3,000 additional people migrated out. As adaptive alternatives become limited because of land scarcity, people often liquidate their vulnerable assets to invest in strategies outside their villages and engage in a more permanent form of migration.

It is the climate vulnerability which makes the Himalayan region an important area of study. The Western Himalayan states are mostly dependent on agriculture and tourism, as discussed in this section. The COVID-19 pandemic and the ensuing lockdown greatly impacted the Indian economy as the country's GDP shrank by 7.3% with millions of jobs and livelihoods at stake. The crisis came at a time when the Indian economy was already slowing down, with unemployment on the rise owing to weak economic performance over the last several years (Dev and Sengupta 2020). The Indian economy, even before the pandemic, was witnessing a demand slowdown which translated into both demand and supply disruptions after the lockdown, impacting both the formal and the informal sectors. Like every state of the country, the Western Himalayan states saw their own pandemic-related economic problems, which are discussed in the next section.

10.3 COVID-19 and the Western Himalayan Region of India

When the COVID-19 pandemic hit the Indian economy with the rest of the world, migrant workers saw themselves at the heart of the plight. As the economy closed down, the fear of job loss and the fear of the virus pushed millions of migrants into distress as a reverse trend of migration started. Most of India's migrant workers come from states like Uttar Pradesh, Bihar, Rajasthan, Madhya Pradesh, Odisha, Jharkhand, West Bengal, and the hill districts of the Himalayan states. An estimated 12 million migrants returned to their places of origin during the initial period of the pandemic. The number of migrants who returned to Uttarakhand during the pandemic was estimated to be about 2.15 lakhs.

Economists have discussed how the return of migrants has led to massive strain on labour supply in urban areas (Dev and Sengupta 2020). However, the impact of such a return was equally faced in the places of origin—mostly, the rural areas. National Sample Survey (NSS) data reveals that the share of rural households reporting out-migration is the highest in the Western Himalayan states. While 30% of rural households in India have reported out-migration according to 2007–08 NSS data, this share is the second highest for Himachal Pradesh (50%) (Kumar 2020). The share of rural households that have reported out-migration is 41% for Uttarakhand. In fact, both Himachal and Uttarakhand have the highest propensity of male out-migration, despite being smaller states in terms of land size (propensity of male out-migration in HP is 2.3 times the national average while it is 1.9 times the national average for Uttarakhand). Studies have also found that migration in Uttarakhand is mostly interstate and is further characterized by low intrastate migration, showing disparities in regional development (Kumar 2020). With low per capita income in the state, rural households are often dependent on remittances as a source of income.

Migration is also gendered and dependent on caste/tribe, religious, and regional identities. As the Indian economy witnessed structural transformation post-liberalization, the labour market became more informal. Migrant groups are often forced into neo-bondage and precarious employment because of continuous debt and brokerage at different phases of the migration process. Caste and class hierarchies, landlessness, meagre wages, lack of adequate work, lack of skills, partial mechanization of farm production, and debt shape the socio-economic and political positions of migrants (Rajan and Sumeetha 2020).

The URDMC interviewed 59,360 reverse migrants from 10 hill districts of Uttarakhand who had returned to their villages from different parts of the country and the world. Many of these returnee migrants belong to the ghost villages or villages which are not inhabited by a single person but whose land and houses are still there. The report found that three hill districts witnessed the largest number of migrants returning due to COVID-19—Pauri, Almora, and Tehri. These are the same three districts which have the largest number of ghost villages among the hill districts of Uttarakhand. Thirty percent of the returnees mentioned that they were willing to stay back if they found proper livelihood opportunities in their villages.

While states like Uttarakhand sees benefit in retaining the returnee migrants, the challenge that these states faced was to accommodate the returnee migrants. Since most of the migrants left their villages in search of livelihood or because of climate change-related issues, the problem for the state was to relocate these returnee migrants and to continue the battle against the climate crisis.

10.3.1 The Role of the State

During any disaster, the state always has a role to play. When the pandemic struck, the Uttarakhand government restricted the entry of all tourists into the state. This implied a massive shock to the people who are dependent on tourism in the state. But the states also took initiatives in distributing food and other essential supplies in many districts of the region.

The major issue, as discussed previously in this book, was accommodating the returnee migrants and providing employment to them. Self-employment was promoted and self-entrepreneurship was seen as a means to this end. The URDMC also recommended access to information related to government schemes and opportunities and providing financial support to encourage self-employment in the travel-tourism and micro-enterprise sectors. A special resettlement package for every migrant was also recommended, in addition to ensuring that basic facilities such as water, school, health centre, and road are built in the resettled ghost villages.

The case of Himachal Pradesh can be highlighted here. The *Mukhyamantri Shahri Ajeevika Guarantee Yojana* (MMSAGY) was started by the HP government in May 2020 with the twin aim of provision of livelihood security and urban asset creation. The MMSAGY guarantees 120 days of wage employment to every household residing in a ULB area and has an annual outlay of Rs 100 crore. Other provisions of the scheme include skill training under the National Urban Livelihood Mission for workers who complete a minimum of 30 days of employment and an unemployment allowance if the worker does not receive work within 15 days of applying. The wage rate—Rs 300 per day—is pegged to the notified minimum wage for urban areas in the state. Although the government has decided to continue with the scheme, it must be noted that its annual outlay has been massively cut to Rs 5 crore from Rs 100 crore in the previous years.

Along with MGNREGA, the MMSAGY in Himachal has successfully provided employment to precarious workers in the state. Rural workers were not the only ones at risk, urban workers were also hit hard during the lockdown. However, the implementation of the scheme has been far from satisfactory. In a research conducted by Choragudi (2022), it was found that many of the workers had not received any work even a year after applying. Some of those who got work—typically for less than 60 days—had to wait one to two months to receive their full wages. According to the data from the Directorate of Urban Development, Government of Himachal Pradesh, the percentage of registered workers accepting work has seen a steady increase since its inception, from 55% in 2020–21 to 75% in 2022–23. However, the percentage of days of work received by each worker on an average has been falling continuously, from 44% in 2020–21 to 19% in 2022–23. This implies that as of January 2022–23, only 19% of the guaranteed days of work, that is, 23 days out of 120 guaranteed days, were provided on average (Chorgudi 2023). Moreover, the workers were not unaware of the unemployment allowance and skill training provisions of the MMSAGY, even though they expressed interest in acquiring skills such as masonry.

Similarly, the Uttarakhand State Government launched the Mukhyamantri Swarojgar Yojana in May 2020 to create employment opportunities for returning migrants. The scheme aimed to provide 15%–25% investment subsidies to returning migrants who wanted to start new services, businesses, and micro-industries for self-employment. However, despite the state government's initiative, more than 1 lakh migrants returned to cities after the pandemic situation improved.

One of the returnee migrants that I interacted with said that it was very difficult to get a loan under the scheme. Another one told me about the endless bureaucracy, paperwork and non-cooperation by banking officials. "Nobody gives any information," said Raghav, a returnee from Gurgaon who had planned to start his own business but gave up on it. Moreover, there is an added challenge of banks requiring collateral to disburse loans. Those who did manage to get a loan found it hard to sustain their businesses against already established players in the domain.

The pandemic reflected the abysmal state of public health of the region as well as the failure of the state to accommodate the returnee migrants and the young people who had lost their livelihoods in one of the most vulnerable regions in the world, which further exacerbated the region's challenges. But stories emerged of how communities took up adaptive measures to combat these challenges.

When I interacted with various communities of the region through civil society bodies, what I found was the building of community resilience as a form of response to the pandemic as the state failed to intervene. This chapter is an attempt to capture narratives and explore the experiences of Western Himalayan communities to understand how the COVID-19 pandemic has affected the lives of people living in a region battling climate change, water crisis, and natural disasters in the midst of the pandemic and how the communities have responded to these challenges.

The method I used was qualitative research through the use of plenary discussions, interviews, and focus group discussions. My research was completely digital since it was done during the peak pandemic in 2020. Through narratives and interpretative phenomenological techniques, a context-specific examination of the respective experiences of these communities before and during the pandemic was attempted. These narratives were constructed by communities in Himachal Pradesh (Spiti and Kanga), Uttarakhand (Bageshwar, Nainital, Almora, Mussoorie, Jhilmil, Munsiyari, and Pauri), Ladakh (Leh, Hanupatta, Meru, Himya, and Lamayuru), and Kashmir (Ganderbam and Srinagar). Interviews and focus group discussions were conducted with local women, youth, and the members of civil society bodies.

10.4 Community Resilience in the Western Himalayas

Past literature has focused on how globalization, climate change, and unequal economic growth have caused difficult or stressful situations like wars, epidemics, natural or human-created disasters, or social inequality for individuals and communities. The term resilience is used by scholars and experts to refer to the adaptive and health-related responses that individuals and groups present when confronted with challenges (Fleming and Ledogar 2008). There is an increasing rise in this group of literature as many of these challenges affect a group of community which share a common definition. Psychological resilience at an individual level was a theme of study in the early 1990s. The focus then gradually shifted to ecology (Oliveira and de Morias 2019).

The initial literature on community resilience was first based on the Latin American context on populations defined by poverty and discrimination, with interventions focused on the social meaning, since the continent is prone to different disasters, stemming from the geographic and social conditions. Ojeda et al. (2018) acknowledges the damage suffered by the community when there is a disaster or catastrophe, but emphasizes that this painful situation can also mean mobilizing the resources and solidarity-creating capabilities of the population to promote physical and social transformations in the community (Oliveira and de Morias 2019). It is as if the communities had a "protective shield," which emerges from their own living conditions and values and allows for the metabolization of a negative event and the possibility of building from it. Through the evaluation of resilience in several communities that suffered disasters, the author observed the conditions that appear more frequently in those that overcome the danger with more rapidity and success and identified the pillars of community resilience, namely solidarity, state honesty, cultural identity, collective self-esteem, and social humour (Oliveira and de Morias 2019). Solidarity is perceived as adherence to the group cause, with the purpose of overcoming adversities and gaining benefits common to all. State honesty is seen as the trust of community members that their governors manage the "public affairs" honestly and transparently. Cultural identity refers to the recognition and appreciation of what is proper to a particular culture, including customs, values, dances, songs, and idiomatic expressions, which gives members a sense of belonging. Social humour is understood as the ability of some people to find comedy in their own tragedy, a strategy that contributes to the acceptance of common misfortune, favouring a distancing from the problem and enabling its resolution. Collective self-esteem refers to an individual's attitude and sense of pride in the place where they live, including a love for their land, awareness of its natural beauty, and identification with certain significant human customs and productions.

According to Norris et al. (2008), community resilience is the process that links a network of adaptive capabilities (resources with dynamic attributes) of a community to a positive trajectory of functionality and adaptation after a disturbance or adversity. The result of the resilience process is community adaptation, manifested by the well-being of the population, which can be defined as high and non-disparate levels of mental and behavioural health, proper functioning of the various social roles and quality of life (how people generally feel about their lives as a whole). This definition links the concept of resilience to traditional concerns in the field of public health and mental health.

As the pandemic changed lives in the region, I tried to understand the role of community resilience in the Western Himalayan states. Climate change research has seen a focus in the rise of community based involvement in the recent years where community resilience plays an important role. Similarly, community-based resilience in times of crisis has been an important part of resilience.

Through a focus on community narratives, I attempted to understand how the COVID-19 pandemic has affected the lives of people living in a region battling climate change, water crisis, and natural disasters in the midst of the pandemic and how the various communities have responded to these challenges. The role of the development sector and non-government organizations is an important highlight of such a response.

10.4.1 Battling Water Crisis (Spring Recharge—Himachal and Uttarakhand)

One major impact of climate change in the Himalayan states of Himachal Pradesh and Uttarakhand is an increase in precipitation events and longer drought periods. Agriculture in the Western Himalayas is to a large extent dependent on spring water. According to data, in the Indian Himalayas, 64% of irrigated areas are fed by springs. However, recent studies have indicated the importance of developing an improved understanding of the aquifers through which groundwater recharges springs (Mahamuni and Kulkarni 2012). Spring discharge is reported to decline due to increased water demand, land use change, and ecological degradation, deforestation, grazing, and exploitative land use resulting in soil erosion and climate change in the Western Himalayan region. With climate change and rising temperatures, rise in rainfall intensity, reduction in its temporal spread, and a marked decline in winter rain, the problem of dying springs is being increasingly felt across the Indian Himalayan Region and threatens whole ways of life for local communities in most parts of the mid-hills of the region.

The level of water of local springs has remained low in many districts of Uttarakhand. There is enough research on how water crisis implies added burden on women as they are the ones who have to fetch water from far-off places. The effects of climate change are always gendered and a shortage of water particularly means more labour work for the womenfolk. “Summers have always been the most difficult season as all the springs dry up and we have to fetch water from far off places,” said Anjali Devi, 38, a resident of Bhalech village in Shimla district of Himachal Pradesh. She also added that a lot of it was because of climate change. “Rainfall used to keep the water in the springs recharged earlier. Nowadays, it is either flood in the monsoon when the water moves downstream rapidly or there is a drought with dry springs.”

As the water crisis has become more acute in the region, the call for the revival of springs and management of these resources have become more urgent and louder. The role of civil society organizations in this is important to highlight as organizations like Central Himalayan Rural Action Group

(CHIRAG), Centre for Ecology Development and Research (CEDAR), and People's Science Institute (PSI) are working to empower local communities to take up sustainable land management, rejuvenate their springs, and raise awareness about the water crisis. Organizations like PSI are mobilizing local women and are providing training for spring rejuvenation (Vikalp Sangam 2021). CHIRAG has trained local communities in creating recharge structures like contour trenches, deep pits, and percolation pits. Rainwater gets collected in these pits during the monsoon and gets soaked into the aquifer. This process further helps in local vegetation.

In the hill districts of Uttarakhand, namely, Pauri, Garhwal, Nainital, Pithoragarh, and Almora, information by the community on which areas need revival and community mobilization played an important role in battling the water crisis. Street theatres or *nukkar nataks* and folk songs sung in local languages helped in creating awareness about spring revival. Locals are then asked if springs need to be revitalized to reduce water scarcity.

The women also prune pine trees to naturally collect the rainwater. "We work in groups," said Nisha Devi, 41, from Nathuakhan village in Nainital district of Uttarakhand, "We prune the trees and remove the weeds. This creates space to plant more trees and preserve the vegetation as well." Water management in the household has primarily been a women's responsibility and thus the burden of water scarcity is eventually felt by women. "We do feel like we are contributing in protecting the environment," Nisha Devi further added.

With efforts from civil society bodies, women have played an important role in rejuvenating springs and mitigating the water crisis in the region. With community involvement of women in the process of spring rejuvenation, it has been a step towards providing agency to women. However, as per Singh (2021), only a few of the villages of the region have shown high female participation in the process. The villages which have indeed seen female participation see very few women participating in the decision-making process.

10.4.2 Returnee Migrants—Ladakh and Uttarakhand

When the pandemic hit the Western Himalayan region of India, a strange phenomenon of reverse migration started happening as migrants started returning back to their villages. The lockdown posed unprecedented challenges for migrants across the world. Migrant workers in different parts of India saw a rise in their vulnerability as many were forced to return to their places of origin. As seen earlier in the chapter, Uttarakhand has seen a high rise in migration over the years. The lockdown saw a loss of almost three-fourths of the migrant workers of the state in Delhi (Mehta 2023).

As migrant workers lost their jobs, returning to their places of origin became a viable option for most. "I had to go back home, there was no job, and I could not keep living with my past savings," said Ankur Bisht, 28, from

Bageshwar. Ankur felt that he could use his savings in investing in something at his hometown rather than spending all the money in a different city.

Although the exact number of return migrants is difficult to estimate, it is claimed that an approximately 2.15 lakh migrants returned to Uttarakhand during the lockdown. Accommodating the returnee migrants became a major issue at the policy level. Different state governments initiated different measures to accommodate the returnee migrants. There was also a different approach by different state governments. The Uttarakhand government was extremely enthusiastic about the returnees given the history of depopulation and "ghost villages" in the state.

As shown in Table 10.3, the districts with the highest returnee migrants are Pauri and Almora. My interviews with 10 returnee migrants of the state reflect data from most government sources—more than 50% of the returnees were employed in the hotel and restaurant industry in the metro cities. My interviews also revealed that the returnees wanted to start their own business or take up entrepreneurship. According to the Interim report, 70% of the returnee migrants were unwilling to work under the Mahatma Gandhi National Employment Guarantee Act (MGNREGA).

Self-employment and entrepreneurship have been celebrated as the solution to the problem of the reverse migrants. But my interviews reveal that lack of awareness about what entrepreneurial venture to pursue, lack of funds or savings for investment, and lack of information on self-employment schemes of the government make the young returnees hesitant in pursuing entrepreneurship. Approaching banks, the unending paperwork and rudeness of officials are some more reasons for credit difficulty amongst the returnees.

Table 10.3 Number of reverse migrants in Uttarakhand during the nationwide lockdown

Name of the District	*Number of Returnee Migrants*	*Percentage of Returnee Migrants*
Almora	43784	20.28
Nainital	9650	4.47
Pithoragarh	5451	2.53
Champawat	15097	6.99
Bageshwar	1925	0.89
Udham Singh Nagar	21958	10.17
Pauri	60440	28.00
Chamoli	5877	2.72
Dehradun	2254	1.04
Haridwar	3136	1.45
Uttarkashi	19405	8.99
Tehri	19242	8.91
Rudraprayag	7656	3.55
Total	215875	100.00

Source: Interim Report of Rural Development & Migration Commission, 20 June 2020

I also spoke to eight returnee migrants in Ladakh. I found a clear distinction in the aspirations of the reverse migrants of Ladakh as compared to those of Uttarakhand. Young female reverse migrants in Ladakh talked more about taking up handicraft and sustainable agriculture. "After I came back home during the lockdown, I had no idea what I should do," said Pangmo, 26, from Ladakh. Pangmo used to work in a mall in Delhi and her return home left her with nothing but her savings. "So, I decided to get into agriculture," Pangmo said, "I started cultivating vegetables in our land." Pangmo's idea of cultivation was not to cater just her, but she cultivated for more households in her neighbourhood. She took help from her neighbours and together they have come up with a sustainable and community agricultural practice. Returnee migrants in Uttarakhand were also keen on taking up agriculture or agro-business activities.

Environmentally sustainable tourism has also been seen as an alternative to commercial tourism. Many of the young people I have talked to did mention about starting their own tourism ventures but in a more sustainable and eco-friendly way. "Uttarakhand is known to attract tourists almost all around the year," said Ramesh Bisht, 24, Pithoragarh. Ramesh has come back to his hometown after completing his graduation and one year of job in Mumbai. "But the need of the hour is when things become normal, we should devise a way to continue tourism here but in a socially and climatically viable way." Like Ramesh, several of my interviewees gave similar response to starting their own tourism ventures.

Birding and avi-tourism are other such ideas that young people, both returnee migrants and the ones who never left their places of origin, are thinking of working on. The United Nations Environment Agency has also recognized that birding can play a significant role in the tourism industry along with its various direct and indirect economic benefits for local communities of developing countries. Irfan Jeelani, 32, from Kangan in Ganderbam district of Kashmir started his own avi-tourism venture called Birds of Kashmir (BOK). But Jeelani's idea soon turned into a community resilience measure against the lockdown. With the idea to attract birdwatchers and familiarize avifauna with the tourists, Jeelani also generated livelihood in an eco-friendly and sustainable way. Now with more than 4,000 members, BOK seeks to create a platform for young people to showcase their own work and become successful professionals in the area. BOK also trains young people in birding and avi-tourism, with the idea of creating a ripple effect in eco-tourism.

This model is not a new one. Many civil society organizations have adopted this model of eco-tourism and training of young people to take up sustainable tourism ventures in the Western Himalayas. With local knowledge about the ecology and knowledge-transfer, sustainable forms of livelihood can be and were created in the Western Himalayan region during the pandemic and the lockdown.

10.5 Conclusion

The COVID-19 pandemic, described as a Black Swan event, created an unprecedented and unpredictable impact on livelihoods of millions of people. The pandemic-induced lockdown led to both market and state failures. The role of the state became central in this neoliberal era of our world—a shift from how we had been living our lives earlier. As Susan Strange puts it, the "retreat of the State"—privatization and contraction of public services and welfare services during the neoliberal globalization of economies became the norm. However, contrary to a financial crisis which requires state intervention in only a particular sector, the pandemic implied a crisis where the state had a major role to play in multiple sectors.

Different governments responded to the crisis differently. The mass migration that India saw took the entire world by shock. Overnight, migrants who had built the cities became homeless in those very cities. Agamben (2020) argued that governments used the pandemic as an opportunity to normalize a state of exception and this state being one with suspension of law and provision of constitutional rights of citizens. Migrants became displaced. People lost jobs. Food became scarce. Agamben further claims that the pandemic gave governments an opportunity to instil fear, curtail movements, deny access to institutions, and suspend the activities of everyday life. Citizens ceased to become rights-bearing individuals.

The Western Himalayan region of the country, with its dependency on tourism and agriculture, saw itself in a peculiar position. When the lockdown hit, the tourism industry faced the highest brunt. But the region also faced a high level of emigration even before the pandemic because of its excessive dependence on agriculture, which remains highly vulnerable to the impact of high climate change in the region. The two factors led to an unprecedented situation in the region. On the one hand, people lost livelihoods as the tourism industry came to a halt. On the other hand, migrants returned to their places of origin. The burden on the state to accommodate the youth who lost jobs in the pandemic and the returnee migrants became the biggest challenge of the region.

When the state failed, the community tried to be more resilient. A region battling climate crisis, the need for sustainable tourism, community-based agriculture, and conservation of natural ecology became the response of the community.

Note

1 Names changed (names of all the respondents have been changed).

References

Agamben, G. 2020. The invention of an epidemic. *The European Journal of Psychoanalysis*. www.journal-psychoanalysis.eu/coronavirus-and-philosophers/

Asian Development Bank. 2010. Annual report 2010 volume 1. www.adb.org/sites/default/files/institutional-document/31388/adb-ar2010-v1.pdf.

Badiger, S., Gopalakrishnan, S. and Patil, I. 2014. Contextualizing rural-urban water conflicts: Bio-physical and socio-institutional issues of domestic water scarcity. In Narain, V., Gurung, C. G., Chourey, C. J. and Prakash, A. (eds.) *Globalization of Water Governance in South Asia*. New Delhi: Routledge Publishers, 204–21.

Bardsley, D. K. and Hugo, G. J. 2010. Migration and climate change: Examining Thresholds of change to guide effective adaptation decision-making. *Population & Environment* 32 (2–3): 238–62.

Black, R., Bennett, S. R. G., Thomas, S. M. and Beddington, J. R. 2011. Climate change: Migration as adaptation. *Nature* 478 (7370): 447–49.

Choragudi, K. P. 2022. Examining Himachal's urban employment guarantee. *Ideas for India*, 21 March 21. www.ideasforindia.in/topics/poverty-inequality/examining-himachal-s-urban-employment-guarantee.html.

Chorgudi, K. P. 2023. Himachal Pradesh: Urban poor families still have a long way to go to get guaranteed employment. *The Wire*, 25 March. https://thewirehindi-com.translate.goog/243574/himachal-pradesh-mukhya-mantri-shahri-ajeevika-guarantee-yojna/?_x_tr_sl=hi&_x_tr_tl=en&_x_tr_hl=en&_x_tr_pto=sc.

Das, L. and Meher, J. K. 2019. Drivers of climate over the Western Himalayan region of India: A review. *Earth Science Reviews* 198.

Dev, S. M. and Sengupta, R. 2020. Covid-19: Impact on the Indian economy. In *Indira Gandhi Institute of Development Research, Mumbai Working Papers 2020–2013*. Mumbai: Indira Gandhi Institute of Development Research.

Dimri, A. P., Chevuturi, A., Niyogi, D., Thayyen, R. J., Ray, K., Tripathy, S. N., Pandey, A. K. and Mohanty, U. C. 2017. Cloud bursts in Indian Himalayas: A review. *Earth Science Reviews* 168: 1–23.

Everitt, A. 1977. River and world: Reflections on the historical origin of regions and pays. *Journal of Historical Geography* 3: 12–20.

Fleming, J. and Ledogar, R. J. 2008. Resilience, an evolving concept: A review of literature relevant to aboriginal research. *Pimatisiwin* 6 (2): 7–23.

Gergan, M. D. 2016. *Precarity and Possibility at the Margins: Hazards, Infrastructure, and Indigenous Politics in Sikkim, India*, unpublished PhD dissertation, The University of North Carolina.

India Brand Equity Foundation. 2022. Himachal Pradesh State Report. September. www.ibef.org/states/himachal-pradesh.

Integrated Mountain Initiative. 2019. 2019–20 Annual Report—VI. https://inmi.in/images/IMI_Annual_report_VI_2019-20.pdf.

Kumar, N. 2020. Diversification of household labour. In Rajan, S. I. and Sumeetha, M. (eds.) *Handbook of Internal Migration*. New Delhi: Sage Publications, 220–34.

Longstaff, P. H., et al. 2010. Building resilient communities: A preliminary framework for assessment. *Homeland Security Affairs* 6, Article 6.

Loria, N. and Bhardwaj, S. K. 2016. Farmers' response and adaptation strategies to climate change in low-hills of Himachal Pradesh in India. *Nature Environment and Pollution Technology an International Quarterly Scientific Journal* 15 (3): 897.

Mahamuni, K. and Kulkarni, H. 2012. Groundwater resources and spring hydrology in South Sikkim, with special reference to climate change. In Arrawatia, M. L. and Tambe, S. (eds.) *Climate Change in Sikkim—Patterns, Impacts, and Initiatives*. Gangtok: Information and Public Relations Department, Government of Sikkim, 261–74.

Mamgain, R. P. and Reddy, D. N. 2017. Out migration from the hill region of Uttarakhand: Magnitude, challenges, and policy options. In Redy, D. N. and Sarap, K. (eds.) *Rural Labour Mobility in Times of Structural Transformation*. Singapore: Palgrave Macmillan, 209–35.

Mehta, B. J. 2023. Migration and Covid-19 pandemic: A study of Uttarakhand migrants in Delhi. *Indian Journal of Human Development* 16 (3): 472.

Mehta, L. 2011. The social construction of scarcity: The case of water in Western India. In Peet, R., Robbins, P. and Watts, M. J. (eds.) *Global Political Ecology*. Routledge, 371–86.

Norri, F. H., et al. 2008. Community resilience as a metaphor, theory, set of capacities, and strategy for disaster readiness. *American Journal of Community Psychology* 41 (1–2): 127–50.

Ojeda, L., Bacigalupe, G., and Pino, A. 2018. Co-production after an urban forest fire: Post-disaster reconstruction of an informal settlement in Chile. *Environment and Urbanization* 30 (2): 537–56. https://doi.org/10.1177/0956247818790731

Oliveira, A. T. C. and de Morias, N. A. 2019. Community resilience: A case study of a community of Fortaleza, CE. *Trends in Psychology* 27 (3): 779–93.

PTI. 2020. Coronavirus impact May render 3.8 crore people jobless in tourism, hospitality sector. *Economic Times*, 19 March. https://economictimes.indiatimes.com/jobs/coronavirus-impact-may-render-3-8-crore-people-jobless-in-tourism-hospitality-sector/articleshow/74709878.cms?from=mdr.

Rahman, A. and Pingali, P. 2024. Development resilience as the scope of social protection. In Rahman, A. and Pingali, P. (eds.) *The Future of India's Social Safety Nets Focus, Form, and Scope*. New York: Palgrave Macmillan, 25–52.

Rajan, S. I. and Sumeetha, M. 2020. Migrant odysseys. In Rajan, S. I. and Sumeetha, M. (eds.) *Handbook of Internal Migration*. New Delhi: Sage Publications, 3–32.

Sangam, V. 2021. *Pandemic Resilience in the Western Himalayas, Volume 3 of the Extraordinary Work of Ordinary People: Beyond Pandemics and Lockdowns*. https://vikalpsangam.org/article/pandemic-resilience-in-the-western-himalayas/

Sati, V. P. 2021. Out-migration in Uttarakhand Himalaya: Its types, reasons, and consequences. *Migration Letters* 18 (3): 285.

Shah, R. 2023. *Disentangling the Drivers of Domestic Water Scarcity in the Eastern Himalayan Region*, unpublished Ph.D. dissertation, Manipal Academy of Higher Education.

Shah, R. and Badiger, S. 2020. Conundrum or paradox: Deconstructing the spurious case of water scarcity in the Himalayan region through an institutional economics narrative. *Water Policy* 22 (S1): 146–61.

Singh, D. V. 1993. A study of impact of agricultural support land on hill economy of Himachal Pradesh. *Indian Journal of Agricultural Economics* 48 (3): 551.

Singh, M. 2021. Spring revival project offers hope amid climate change in the Himalayas. *The Third Pole*, 26 August. www.thethirdpole.net/en/livelihoods/springs-uttarakhand-project-climate-change-himalayas/.

Tacoli, C. 2009. Crisis or adaptation? Migration and climate change in a context of high mobility. *Environment and Urbanization* 21 (2): 513.

Terbek, C. C. H. 2014. Impacts of climate change on mountains. *UNESCO*, 3 December. www.unesco.org/en/articles/mountains-provide-early-warning-climate-change#:~:text=The%20exhibition%20'Climate%20change%20impacts,key%20indicators%20of%20climate%20change.

World Bank. 2012. *Turn Down the Heat: Why a 4°C Warmer World Must be Avoided*. Washington, DC: World Bank.

Wrathall, D. J., Bury, J., Carey, M., Mark, B., McKenzie, J., Young, K., Baraer, M., French, A. and Rampini, C. 2013. Migration amidst climate rigidity traps: Resource politics and social–ecological possibilism in Honduras and Peru. *Annals of the Association of American Geographers* 10 (3): 1–13.

For Product Safety Concerns and Information please contact our EU representative GPSR@taylorandfrancis.com
Taylor & Francis Verlag GmbH, Kaufingerstraße 24, 80331 München, Germany

www.ingramcontent.com/pod-product-compliance
Lightning Source LLC
LaVergne TN
LVHW021128300926
849160LV00010B/905
* 9 7 8 1 0 3 2 9 6 9 9 8 5 *